KETOGENIC DIET

What to Eat While Losing Weight

Table of contents

Introduction

I want to thank you and congratulate you for downloading the book, *"Ketogenic Diet: What to Eat While Losing Weight"*.

This book contains proven steps and strategies on how to successfully eat healthier, lose weight and achieve optimum health through an effective and safe method—the ketogenic diet.

The number of overweight and obese individuals is increasing in an alarming rate. More and more individuals are also experiencing negative self-body image brought about the excess weight, some may even have several health issues that are affecting their quality of living or is just plain detrimental and even has economic downside.

Some of the most common health complications of being overweight are:

- Cardiovascular diseases
- Type2 Diabetes
- Stroke
- Osteoarthritis
- Sleep apnea
- High blood pressure
- Cancer (colon, breast, kidney, esophagus and more)
- Gout
- Gallbladder disease and gallstones

Taking into consideration the physical, mental, social and psychological impact of our weight has on our whole being, proper weight management is must.

Being healthy is an everyday choice that you should make. There are hundreds of diet regimens available, exercise routines, medical procedures, and even diet supplements that are sold in the market, and sometimes it gets confusing on what you follow. Some can be effective, others may produce a yo-yo effect, and others are more damaging that beneficial. Your goal should be an effective diet that has an overall positive impact on your health.

What you need is not just changing what you eat, but also changing your mindset that you will take certain course of actions that are healthy and nurturing for your body. This is where the ketogenic diet will come in. It is proven safe and effective and is viable for a complete lifestyle change. You will be embracing a high-fat, adequate-protein, low-carbohydrate diet that will absolutely change your life!

Warning, this can be entirely different from the way that you used to eat, but it will be worth it to take the extra effort of planning and choosing your meals properly. How does achieving your target body weight sounds to you? Being able to wear what you want? Having the chance to play with your kids without losing your breath because you are now absolutely healthy? Do you want to have that extra boost on your self-confidence? Or just simply feel good about yourself? You can achieve all of those with ketogenic diet.

Make the decision now to start with the ketogenic diet, and I guarantee you, this will be one of the best health decisions that you will ever make. Hundreds have already attained their health goals with this lifestyle change and you can do it too.

Do not fret, this book contains helpful tips on how to start your diet, what to eat and what not to eat, address common pitfalls and more. I will also be throwing in a sample meal plan to jumpstart your diet! All you have to is make that decision and commit to a better and healthier you.

Thanks again for downloading this book, I hope that you will not only enjoy it but will also help you in your weight loss and get-healthy journey!

CHAPTER 1:

Basic Ketogenic Diet Information

What most people do not realize is that before embarking on any diet regimen, you have to first understand how your body works, or how your system will process the food intake. Some will just cut down their carbs, fats or any deemed junk foods, but in reality, if you want the diet regimen to be really efficient and be able to reap its maximum benefits, you have to understand the quality of food intake, proper type of food to consume and sometimes even the right portioning.

For fitness junkies, ketogenic diet is actually one of the most popular diets in the low-calorie world. But unlike any other low-cal diets, there is a definite percentage on the types of food that you should consume.

So how does it work?

We all know that we need food for energy. On a typical high-carb diet, our body specifically uses glucose as the primary source of energy since it is easier to convert compared with other types of energy source (from carbs to glucose). Insulin will also be produced by the body to process the glucose in our blood stream, and the fats in our body will just be stored and will eventually pile up.

Ketogenic diet introduces another energy source to fuel the needs of our body.

The concept is that with lower carb intake, you will be depriving your body of the glucose it needs, and will make use of the fats instead, as it falls into a state known as ketosis.

Ketosis is actually a natural state of the body wherein the liver will breakdown the available fats instead of glucose or carbs, and ketones will be produced, which will be burned by the body as the energy source.

Your goal with ketogenic diet is to *force* your body into this metabolic state. You don't have to worry about this since our bodies are designed to easily adapt to this state.

I would also like to stress that ketogenic diet is different from other low carbohydrate diets. The difference is that your diet should be about 70-75% of calories from fat, 20-25% from protein and 5-10% from carbohydrate on a daily basis. This means that your diet will be composed of high-fats and moderate protein intake. No need to count the calories.

If you'll notice, protein is also limited because of the reason that protein also affects the insulin and blood sugar of the body. If consumed in large quantities, the excess will also be converted to glucose. In effect, your body will not reach the state of ketosis

In addition, have you observed that whenever you have a certain food craving, you usually go for carb-rich foods? That's because our brains has "labeled" the starchy and sweet foods as "comfort food". Our main goal in this diet is to drastically reduce this sinful food category, and choose a healthier alternative. In theory, if we limit one's carbohydrate intake, and achieve that state of ketosis, the excess weight will be shed easily.

How did the ketogenic diet start?

Invented by Dr. Russell Wilder, the ketogenic diet has been around for about 90 years. Before becoming a well-known diet in the fitness world, it was first introduced as an effective treatment for epilepsy like Lennox-Gastaut syndrome (mostly used for children). When anti-seizure medications were invented in the 1940s, it soon fell out of fashion. It returned to the spotlight in 1994 because it was used in the case of a son of a Hollywood producer who has epilepsy Charlie Abrahams, who showed improvement after following the ketogenic diet.

Charlie's case, sparked interest in health professionals to do more research and propagate the diet.

By the year 2007, the diet was then available in 45 countries and was known to not only improve epilepsy but also the condition of patients with cancer, autism, Alzheimer's among others.

A few years ago, it was found out that the diet could also curb the appetite and promote weight loss. That's why in recent years, the ketogenic diet was used by celebrities like Kim Kardashian and more, which further popularized the diet.

Other Benefits of Ketogenic Diet and Low Carb Diet

- Say goodbye to hunger pangs- this is one of the amazing benefits of a keto diet. Your hunger pangs will be curbed, because you are satiated with the quality and nutritious food that you are consuming. Your body will also have lesser signal cravings for more food volume compared to when you are in a high-carbohydrate diet.
- More beneficial hormones released e.g. growth hormone- this is triggered by the lower level of insulin in the body. As a result, there will free glycerol release and greater lipolysis, as compared with a normal diet.
- Fats are now utilized –when you are in a high-carb diet, your body's fat is actually on a "lazy" state, so with keto, the fats are on the go and is used as fuel instead.
- Weight loss- a low carb diet is one of the most effective ways to lose the extra pounds. In addition, the excess water and excess sodium in the body are flushed out that can lead to rapid weight loss.

- Say goodbye to hypertension -lower blood pressure is another amazing effect of a low carb diet. This also means that the risk for kidney failure, stroke, heart diseases and more are reduced.
- Increase of High Density Lipoprotein (HDL) – "good" cholesterol in the body will increase. The higher your good cholesterol, the lower your risk of heart diseases.

Worries with Ketogenic Diet

Not surprisingly, the most issue for individuals before embarking on the ketogenic diet is their "fear" of fats. For most of us, our minds have been programmed to believe that fats can make you fat and that fat is not good for the health. But in fact, these are unfounded, and the reality is, a high carb diet is actually unhealthier as it can drive up your blood sugar and insulin level, which can cause inflammation in the body that can cause heart diseases and other medical condition.

With ketogenic diet, not only will you lose weight, but the low-carbs and high fats combo can also effectively reduce the risk of developing inflammation-related illnesses. So let go of your fears, ketogenic diet is proven safe and effective.

Can Everyone Try the Ketogenic Diet?

Your overall health should be of the utmost importance. Just like any diet plans, I suggest that you consult your healthcare provider especially if you have the following health problems:

- Gastric bypass surgery
- History of pancreatitis and kidney failure

- Impaired liver function
- Heart problems
- Abdominal tumors
- Impaired fat digestion
- Poor nutritional status
- Active gall bladder disease

Now that we know how the diet works, and if you are excited to reap its weight loss and health benefits, let's now get started with the diet!

CHAPTER 2

How to Start a Ketogenic Diet

As soon as you make that decision that you want to start with the ketogenic diet, the next step to make is to of course start the preparation process. Like any journey that you have to make, preparation is one of the keys to success. I also have to warn you that dieting is not just a physical battle, but is of the mind. You will be tempted with your "comfort" food, tantalized by your cravings, or there would be days that you feel like it's harder to follow your lifestyle change. But the key here is self-control and achieving a healthy state of mind and the body.

To help you jumpstart the diet, here are the first few things that you should do:

✓ Research! You most likely heard that knowledge is power, and this is indeed true even in dieting. You need to get all the information that you can that will help you with the dieting process. This book will provide the necessary information to help you start the diet, but there are more materials that you can explore like ketogenic cookbooks and more.

✓ Goal-setting – you have to set tangible goals, which can give you the extra boost that you need to succeed. Do not just say "I want to lose weight", you have to be definite and at the same time realistic. For example, "I want to lose 10 pounds in a month, my weekly weight loss should be...." You can list down your food intake and even daily activities so that you can track what you eat. Make sure that you have written down your starting weight and measurements. You can also take photos so that you can compare the changes in your body. As you reach your goal, you can also make new ones. This will give you a sense of accomplishment and will also add to your self-confidence.

✓ Ready your gears- though there is no special diet or tools required for the ketogenic diet, it will be beneficial for you if you will have some "gears" to help you out like ketostix reagent strip (this optional if you want to track your ketone level especially on the first few weeks), helpful apps like food tracker, carb counter guide and more. As they say, you need all the help and reminder that you can get.

✓ Have a support system – it will beneficial if you inform the people that you are usually with, like family members, friends and workmates about your diet, so that they will know that you will be undergoing some lifestyle changes. They will also be more sensitive in offering you food, teasing you to eat and more.

From there, you can also choose an accountability buddy, which will not only support or motivate you but also remind you in times that you may go astray. You can even ask your partner or friend to go through the diet with you and be healthy together! This will make the whole process easier and even more fun plus you can share your food goodies!

✓ Join a keto group- there are actually a lot of keto-related groups that you can join in the social media world. This group can also serve as your support system or can even further guide you and give tips to make the diet easier.

✓ Remember that consistency is the key- you have to understand and internalize that in ketogenic diet, there is no room for "cheat days". This is a commitment that you have to keep. Why? Because if you suddenly consume loads of sweets or carbs, the fat-burning process or the ketosis will be put in halt! You will have to start all over again. But do not worry, there are a lot of delicious recipes to choose from that you might not even miss your old unhealthy food!

✓ Timing is everything- you have probably heard of this saying and this is also especially true in starting your ketogenic diet. Do not just start right away, think about the timing, it is best to try the diet after the big holidays like Christmas or Thanksgiving. Why? There is a lot of rooms for temptations, and since you're in that merry holiday mood, and with some coaxing from your relatives or friends, there is a huge chance that you will give in. Unless you really feel that you have an iron-clad self-control. Do not start until you are fully committed and prepared.

✓ Clear out your pantry and restock- yup, you have to say good bye and let go of all of the unhealthy and non-keto goodies that you have (yes, even your hidden stash). Raid your cupboard and fridge, throw them out, give them out or have your own special corner if you are the only family member that will try the diet. Again, do not put yourself in situations that can tempt you, and that includes opening a cupboard full of chocolates and starchy food. The next step is to prepare yourself a grocery list (I will provide the dos and don'ts on the next chapter) and restock your kitchen. Again, there are no special food items that you buy, but you have to prepare yourself since you are most likely do a lot of cooking or spend some time in your kitchen. Definitely no fast food for you.

✓ No exercise for the first two weeks- with exceptions if you are already fit, I suggest that you skip the exercising for the next two weeks. Why? Your body will be undergoing a lot of changes, especially if you are really unfit, allow it to adjust first to the changes. Do not stress yourself with too many changes at the same time. After the adjustment period you can proceed with an exercise regimen of your choice. If you do have one, you can start with walking for at least 30 minutes a day.

✓ **Love you H2O- as you start this diet, don't forget to drink more water than what you are used to. Why? As you lower your carb intake, your kidney will start disposing the excess water that you have retained. So make sure to drink up to avoid dehydration. You can also add in more minerals with your water intake.**

✓ Learn some techniques to stop sugar cravings- as I have said this is a battle of the mind. Aside from the self-control that you have, it won't hurt if you will have some techniques on hand that will help stop your sugar cravings. Example, as soon as you feel the sugar craving coming in, distract yourself, go for a walk , drinks lots of water or do other tasks until the craving have already subsided.

✓ Consult your doctor – the ketogenic diet is a relatively safe diet, but if you have any pre-existing condition/s then your doctor will be the one to give you the go signal to proceed or not.

✓ Be easy on yourself- you will be replacing your old habits so expect that you will experience some bumps along the road. Give yourself time to adjust, remember that it takes 21 days to replace or create new habits. Don't also expect that all the excess pounds that you have should magically disappear in just a few days, it took one pound at a time to accumulate those, so expect that your body will also need some time to shed those (don't worry it wouldn't be that long with keto diet to see the results!). So be patient and enjoy the process!

CHAPTER 3

What Food to Eat and What to Avoid in Ketogenic Diet

As I have said be prepared to spend some time in the kitchen. If you want your keto diet to work, you have to plan ahead your daily meals. Do not forget this guideline: 70-75% of calories from fat, 20-25% from protein and 5-10% from carbohydrate.

If you want to have a more restrictive diet, you should only restrict your carbs to less than 15g a day to fast track the state of ketosis. In general, most of your carbs should be from nuts, veggies and dairy. You have to stir away from any refined carbs like pastas and bread, even starchy veggies or fruits.

My standard suggestion on meals should be a protein-packed dish with veggies on the side. In case you will feel hungry or starts to crave for food that is on the no-no list, you can start munching on some cheeses, nuts, seeds and my favorite, a spoonful of peanut butter.

1. Your food intake will be mostly from fats (do not forget this mantra "fats are your friends") but you also have to be cautious to take quality fats only. Say no to hydrogenated fats (e.g. margarine) and choose non-hydrogenated lards or coconut oil instead for frying. You should also not use interestified fats like corn oils, canola oils and sunflower oils.

   ✓ Avocado
   ✓ Peanut Butter(choose the unsweetened version)
   ✓ Organic chicken fat
   ✓ Mayonnaise (count the carbs and choose the sugar free version)
   ✓ Avocado oil
   ✓ Beef tallow
   ✓ Butter
   ✓ Olive oil, organic
   ✓ Organic duck fat
   ✓ Organic leaf lard
   ✓ Almond oil
   ✓ Macadamia Nuts
   ✓ Macadamia oil
   ✓ Olives
   ✓ Organic coconut oil
   ✓ Coconut butter
   ✓ Coconut cream concentrate

✓ Seed and most nut oils
✓ Clarified butter
✓ Organic Red Palm oil
✓ Polyunsaturated omega 3s, especially from animal sources

2. **Sources of Protein**

   ✓ Grass-fed meat like lamb, beef, lamb, venison and goat
   ✓ Wild-caught fish & seafood - avoid farmed fish ; try sardines, halibut, salmon, shrimp, mackerel, mahi-mahi tuna, salmon etc.
   ✓ Pastured pork
   ✓ Eggs – preferable organic
   ✓ Poultry- try the free range version
   ✓ Sausages
   ✓ Soy products
   ✓ Sugar free bacon- check out some specialty healthy stores
   ✓ Whey protein powders
   ✓ Peanut butter

3. **Fresh vegetables**-preferably organic are recommended. The best types of veggies are the dark and leafy green vegetables and try to avoid the starchy vegetables and the sweet ones like carrots.

   ✓ Cabbage
   ✓ Swiss chard
   ✓ Kale
   ✓ Bok choy
   ✓ Brussels sprouts
   ✓ Cauliflower

- ✓ Celery
- ✓ Onions
- ✓ Leafy green vegetables
- ✓ Bamboo shoots
- ✓ Broccoli
- ✓ Asparagus
- ✓ Cucumbers
- ✓ Bean sprouts
- ✓ Chives
- ✓ Radishes
- ✓ Garlic
- ✓ Turnips
- ✓ Shallots
- ✓ Spinach
- ✓ Endive
- ✓ Summer squash

Note that in ketogenic diet, fruits are not that recommended because of its high glucose content. You can just consume them occasionally like berries.

4. Dairy products –though allowed, go for the raw or organic milk products. Note: run away from products labeled as "low fat", the reality is that most have some starch and sugar content.

- ✓ Unsweetened whole milk yoghurt
- ✓ Heavy whipping cream
- ✓ Full fat cottage cheese
- ✓ Hard and soft cheeses like mozzarella and cheddar

5. **Spices** – do not worry, your food will definitely not lack flavor. Note that you still have to be careful in the carb content of your spices.

- ✓ Sea salt – choose this over table salt
- ✓ Basil
- ✓ Sage
- ✓ Cinnamon
- ✓ Cilantro
- ✓ Chili pepper
- ✓ Black pepper
- ✓ Turmeric
- ✓ Parsley
- ✓ Peppermint
- ✓ Thyme
- ✓ Cumin seeds
- ✓ Ginger
- ✓ Mustard seeds
- ✓ Rosemary
- ✓ Cayenne pepper

6. **Sweeteners** – some sweeteners are allowed in this diet like:

- ✓ Stevia
- ✓ Monk Fruit
- ✓ Swerve
- ✓ Erythrito

7. **Nuts and Seeds**

- ✓ Almonds
- ✓ Pecans
- ✓ Hazelnuts
- ✓ Flax seed
- ✓ Sunflower seed
- ✓ Pumpkin seed
- ✓ Sesame seed

✓ Brazil nuts (limited intake only due to high level of selenium)
✓ Walnuts
✓ Hemp seeds
✓ Almonds
✓ Pine nuts

8. **Beverages and Alcohols**

✓ Coffee
✓ Tea
✓ Dry red wine
✓ Unsweetened spirits
✓ Dry white wine

The BIG NO NOs – here is a list of food that you should completely avoid. Consuming them will stop the process of ketosis due to their contents.

1. All grains and grain product

✓ Wheat
✓ Oats
✓ Corn
✓ Quinoa
✓ Barley
✓ Rye
✓ Rice
✓ Bread
✓ Pasta
✓ Cereal
✓ Pancakes
✓ Crackers
✓ Cookies

- ✓ Tortillas
- ✓ Muffins
- ✓ Bagels
- ✓ Beers (made from grains)

2. **Sugar and Sweetened Food** –word of caution, you should always read the labels. Familiarize yourself with terms that are actually referring to a form of sugar.

  - ✓ Powdered sugar
  - ✓ Sorghum,
  - ✓ Cane sugar
  - ✓ Maple syrup
  - ✓ Brown sugar
  - ✓ Glucose
  - ✓ Corn syrup
  - ✓ Lactose
  - ✓ Fructose
  - ✓ Maltose
  - ✓ Honey
  - ✓ Candies

3. **Processed food**- these are laden with fillers and preservatives, and even if you are not in a ketogenic diet, ditch these type of food completely.

  1. **Corn products**
     - ✓ Cornbread
     - ✓ Polenta
     - ✓ Popcorn
     - ✓ Corn grits
     - ✓ Corn chips
     - ✓ Corn syrup

4. **Fruit Juices and Diet Sodas**- high sugar content alert! Stick with the water.

In case you will suddenly have some cravings, at times your body is actually just craving for a particular nutrient. Here are some alternatives that you can eat:

- ✓ Chocolates (magnesium) – much on some seeds and nuts
- ✓ Bread and pasta (nitrogen) – replace it with high protein mean. You could also try some "veggie pasta".
- ✓ Salty food- try some dishes out of fish or some nuts can do some wonders.
- ✓ Sugary food (phosphorus, carbon, chromium, tryophan, sulphur)-cheese, spinach, veggies like broccoli, eggs m chicken and more.

Sample meal plan (good for 3-4 days):

Breakfast   full fatGreek yogurt or some almond flour pancakes or be safe with some egg dishes like some omelets.

Lunch   ☐ Classic Tuna Sandwich /

Cauliflower rice and Chicken Cordon Bleu/

Salad greens with cubed ham

Snacks   a slice of avocado / sugar free sausage /nuts / lettuce wraps

Dinner   ☐ Cajur

Knowledge on the right food to eat and self-control is the key if you want to religiously follow the ketogenic diet. What is good with this diet is that you will not go hungry and there are actually hundreds of yummy dishes and alternatives that you can work on.

CHAPTER 4

Common Pitfalls for Keto Newbies

I would not lie to you, like with any diet, sometimes there are a few snags that you might experience. I will be giving you the common pitfalls that I have observed on newbies so that you may avoid them and have an easier ride to weight loss and optimal health. And if in case you will experience this pitfall, just repeat the process!

Again, do not be hard on yourself. Just stand firm on your goal and do your best, you will surely find that the keto diet is fairly doable.

1. Eating too much protein-in ketogenic diet, though protein is allowed, the key is "moderate" amount only.

Most keto dieters consuming lean animal food, if not careful, may consume too much of it. Most of us don't know is that protein can actually turn into glucose through gluconeogenesis. This means that you will be preventing your body to go into full ketosis, thus defeating the purpose of the diet.

2. Not wanting to eat- a low-carb diet is not equivalent to starvation. Or some may even have the wrong notion of not only lowering the carbohydrate intake but also the FAT intake. I will repeat it, FAT is your friend. Besides, if you also reduce your fat intake, where will your body get its energy? Plus you are actually more prone to temptation when you are not satiated and starving. So consume the required amount of fats and proteins, and weight loss will follow.

3. Too many changes – allow yourself to adapt with one change after another. As soon as you are well adjusted to the keto plan, then that's the time that you can adopt a more active lifestyle to further help you in the getting fit process. Be patient and be kind to your body.

4. Not replacing electrolytes and not increasing the amount of water intake – do not forget that with this diet the water in your body is expelled quickly and your electrolytes are actually excreted through your urine. The key is constant replenishment. If not, then you will be most likely be down with "ketoflu", which is characterized with nausea, headaches, upset stomach, fatigue, brain fog and more. A lot of newbies will think that keto is making them sick and is unhealthy so they will stop with the diet. But the truth is, the lack of water and electrolytes are causing the sickness. So drink plenty

of water and take some supplements. You could also try some coconut water or some healthy broth to replace the lost electrolytes.

5. Giving up on the diet because of some fat adaptation symptoms-some may experience a metallic after-taste in their mouth, some sudden burst of energy, or will notice that their pee has a different smell, again, do not worry. This is normal. Also, you have to allow your body to adapt, and even if you are not feeling that well at first, your body will soon regulate and will start using those stored fats as energy.

6. Cheating–do not fool yourself. Cheating is not allowed with ketogenic diet. Instead, I encourage you to find alternatives to soothe your cravings. You might wonder why is the diet taking too long, but have forgotten those sneaky chocolate bars and strawberry cakes that you've been eating in "small portions" a day. You have to fully commit in order to see the positive outcomes.

As you are reading this, you might think that you are required to do a lot, but in reality, these are only small discomforts that you should endure in exchange of the body that you want plus being able to eliminate various health risks. Even in other types of diets, there are also rules or things that you should do. If you really want to succeed, which you can, then exert the necessary effort. A lot of people were able to this diet. So can you!

CHAPTER 5:

Ketogenic Recipes

Breakfasts

Healthy Breakfast Casserole

Ingredients

2 sourdough rolls, cut into cubes

3 Portobello mushroom caps, diced

2 cups egg whites

12 grape tomatoes, cut into thirds

150g fresh spinach, torn

½ red onion, diced

3 red peppers, roasted and peeled

2 yellow potatoes, diced

450g zucchini, sliced

2 tbsp. olive oil

200g ricotta cheese

4 tbsp. pecorino Romano cheese, grated

Directions

Start by setting your oven to 400 degrees F.

Combine the diced onions and the potatoes on a baking sheet and drizzle with half a tsp. of olive oil.

Roast for about fifteen minutes then remove from oven.

Next, drizzle the zucchini with half a tbsp. of olive oil and toss well then add this to the baking sheet. Retune to the oven and bake for about 40 minutes or until the veggies start turning golden.

Meanwhile, sauté the mushrooms in half a tbsp. of olive oil then transfer to a plate. Add the remaining olive oil to the pan and sauté the spinach until wilted.

Now, mix the egg whites with the cheeses in a bowl then set aside.

In a baking dish, combine the cubed sourdough, all veggies and grape tomatoes and stir well to combine. Pour the egg-cheese mixture on top then bake for about 45 minutes. Remove from oven and let stand for 10 minutes before serving.

Enjoy an easy, high protein Mediterranean breakfast!

Yummy Breakfast Stir Fry

Ingredients

2 egg whites, beaten

2 small onions, chopped

2 green peppers, chopped

4 medium tomatoes, chopped

A handful mushrooms, chopped

1 tbsp. extra virgin olive oil, a good pinch of sea salt, or to taste

Black olives, hot banana peppers and sliced cucumber, for serving

Directions

Add olive oil to a pan and add the green peppers. Cover and cook on high heat for about 2 minutes then lower the heat and cook for 3 more minutes.

Next add the onions and the mushrooms and cover. Cook until tender then stir in the tomatoes. Sprinkle the salt, cover and simmer for about 15 minutes or until the melamen is soft and juicy.

Gently drizzle the egg whites over the melamen. Allow to cook without stirring for about a minute.

Roast the hot bananas peppers on your burner over medium heat, careful not burn them too much.

Serve the stir fry with whole wheat pita bread, black olives, roasted hot banana pepper and sliced cucumbers. You can also serve with traditional Mediterranean tea.

Enjoy!

Hearty Breakfast Wrap

Ingredients

2 multi grain flax wraps

3 egg whites

1 ½ tbsp. extra virgin olive oil

¼ cup sun dried tomatoes

¼ cup fresh spinach, chopped

¼ cup crumbled feta cheese

Sea salt and freshly ground pepper to taste

Directions

Heat the oil in a nonstick pan and sauté the tomatoes, spinach and egg whites until almost done then flip and cook the other side.

Add the crumbled feta to warm it up. Sprinkle with salt and pepper then remove from heat.

Heat the wraps on a dry pan then serve the egg mixture into the wraps and roll them up.

Enjoy!

Breakfast Tofu Scramble

Ingredients

450g extra firm tofu, drained and pressed for a minimum of 20 minutes

2 cloves garlic, minced

3 green onions, sliced

1 red onion, diced

1 red pepper, diced

1 tbsp. freshly squeezed lemon juice

2 tbsp. low sodium soy sauce

1 ½ tbsp. za'atar seasoning

2 tbsp. extra virgin olive oil

1 tsp turmeric powder

¼ cup fresh parsley, finely chopped

½ tsp red chili flakes

Pita bread and hot sauce or hummus for serving

Directions

Add olive oil to a large pan over medium heat and sauté the red onions until tender then add in the garlic and cook for 1 more minute.

Gently crumble the tofu into the pan and stir in the red pepper, lemon juice, soy sauce, za'atar and chili flakes. Cook as you stir frequently for about 5 minutes until the red pepper is crisp – tender.

Ketogenic Diet

Turn off the heat and fold in the green onions and the parsley.

Serve with pita bread and hot sauce or hummus if you prefer.

Enjoy!

Breakfast Quesadillas

Ingredients

1 skinned and boneless chicken breast

1 cup fresh baby spinach, torn

2 eggs + 2 egg whites

½ cup tomatoes, seeded and finely chopped

1 avocado, chopped

1 ½ tbsp. extra virgin olive oil

¼ cup black olives, sliced

¼ cup sour cream

1/3 cup shredded cheddar cheese

3 scallions, sliced

3 tbsp. fresh cilantro, finely chopped

Directions

Start by preheating the broiler then pound the breast to make it tender. Season generously with kosher salt and pepper and broil for about 5 minutes until it's no longer pink on the inside. Remove from broiler and transfer to a cutting board and dice it.

Next preheat your oven to 200 F.

Meanwhile, whisk the eggs and egg whites in a medium bowl.

Add a tbsp. of olive oil into a pan over medium heat and pour in the egg mixture. Once the eggs start setting, use a spatula to scrap the eggs on the bottom, folding them towards the center.

Stir in the chicken, tomatoes and spinach and continue cooking until the eggs become light and fluffy then remove from heat.

Add the remaining olive to a separate pan and place it on medium heat then add a tortilla to heat through. The olive oil will make the tortilla crispy and yummy.

Flip over the tortilla and top it with some of the cheese. Add some of the egg mixture as well the fold the tortilla in half and continue cooking until the tortilla starts browning. Follow the same process as you make the remaining quesadillas.

Cut the quesadillas into wedges and top with avocado, scallions, olives, sour cream, cilantro and salsa if you desire.

Enjoy!

Yummy Eggs And Sausage

Ingredients

4 eggs

2 chorizo sausages, chopped

¼ cup Kalamata olives, pitted and coarsely chopped

½ cup bottled roasted red peppers, drained and cut into long strips

1 tbsp. extra virgin olive oil

½ tsp harissa paste

1 tsp brown sugar

1 ¾ cups tomato sauce

1 tbsp. freshly chopped parsley

Multigrain crusty bread for serving

Directions

Add the olive oil to a large pan and fry the sliced sausage until crispy. Stir in the tomato sauce, harissa, sugar and the roasted peppers. Lower the heat once it starts boiling and simmer for 10 minutes then stir in the sliced olives.

Make four wells in the sausage sauce and crack the 4 eggs into each well. Cover the pan and cook for 5 minutes or until the whites set but the yolks remain runny.

Garnish with the chopped parsley and sprinkle with salt and freshly ground pepper if desired. Serve immediately with the crusty bread.

Enjoy!

Yummy Greek Breakfast Bowl

Ingredients

½ cup Greek cucumber, thinly sliced

½ cup unsalted chickpeas, drained

2 Kalamata olives, pitted and sliced

1 ½ tsp extra virgin olive oil

2 tbsp. slivered roasted red bell peppers

1 ½ tsp red wine vinegar

2 tbsp. crumbled feta cheese

A dash of kosher salt

A good pinch of freshly ground black pepper

2 tsp freshly chopped dill

Directions

Combine the olive oil, salt, pepper and vinegar in a medium bowl and whisk well using a fork.

Mix in the chickpeas, olives and bell peppers and toss well to combine.

Arrange the thinly sliced cucumber on a serving bowl and top with the chickpea mixture, crumbled cheese and the chopped dill.

Enjoy!

The Ultimate Breakfast Frittata

Ingredients

4 eggs

150g salami, diced

28g black olives, sliced

750g potatoes, peeled and diced

2 tbsp. extra virgin olive oil

1 small zucchini, diced

1 red onion, cut into rings

1 red onion, diced

5 sprigs basil, finely chopped

1 tsp balsamic vinegar

300g diced tomatoes

1/3 cup whipped cream

Directions

Add half the olive to a large pan over medium to high heat and fry the potatoes for about 12-15 minutes. Stir in the onion rings, olives, zucchini and salami and cook for 5 minutes.

Whisk the eggs and cream and season with salt and pepper then pour over the potato mixture. Cover the pan and cook over medium to low heat for 10 minutes.

Meanwhile, toss the diced onions, tomatoes, basil, the remaining olive oil and vinegar and season well to taste. Cut the frittata into wedges and top with the tomato salad.

Enjoy!

Green Eggs With Ham

Ingredients

8 eggs

8 bacon strips, fried and crumbled

2 tbsp. milk

3 cups cubed potatoes – seasoning (garlic salt, low sodium veggie broth, Spanish paprika and freshly ground black pepper)

¼ cup Kalamata olives, pitted and chopped

3 tbsp. chopped roasted red peppers

2 cups fresh baby spinach

1 tbsp. extra virgin olive oil

¼ cup crumbled bacon

½ tsp kosher salt

Directions

Start by setting your oven to 375 F.

Meanwhile place the potatoes in a mixing bowl and pour in just enough veggie broth to wet the potatoes. Season with garlic salt, black pepper and paprika then arrange the seasoned potatoes on a baking sheet and roast for half an hour or until tender.

Add the olive oil to a large pan over medium heat and sauté the baby spinach until wilted then transfer to a plate.

Beat the eggs together with the milk, salt and pepper in a medium bowl. Spray the large pan with cooking spray and pour in the egg mixture. Scramble the eggs using a rubber spatula but careful not to overcook them.

Stir in the spinach, olives, bacon, roasted peppers and feta cheese until well combined.

To serve, start with the roast potatoes and top with the green eggs.

Enjoy!

Breakfast Chicken Casserole

Ingredients

330g boneless chicken thighs, cubed

4 slices bacon

1 Spanish onion, cut into thin wedges

60g button mushrooms, sliced

1 zucchini, chopped

2 tbsp. extra virgin olive oil

30g black olives, sliced

370g chopped tomatoes with herbs

¼ cup low sodium chicken stock

1 tbsp. flat leaf parsley, finely chopped for garnish

Leftover pasta or crusty bread to serve

Directions

Set your oven to 450 F.

Heat the olive oil in an oven proof pan over medium to high heat and fry the chicken for about 3 minutes or until evenly browned. Transfer the chicken to a plate covered with kitchen towels and add the mushrooms, bacon, onions and zucchini to the pan. Cook for about 5 minutes then add the browned chicken, chicken stock, olives and the herbed tomatoes.

Place the pan in the oven and bake for about half an hour or until the chicken is completely cooked through.

Serve with the leftover pasta or crusty bread.

Enjoy!

Breakfast Torte

Ingredients

2 packages frozen spinach

1 package frozen bread dough

300g marinated red pepper strips

400g artichoke hearts, quartered

450g fresh mushrooms

200g ham, thinly sliced and cooked

200g salami, thinly sliced

1 egg

150g provolone cheese

1 tbsp. water

Directions

Divide the thawed bread dough into two and roll out one part on a floured surface into a wide circle then cover and set aside. Roll out the remaining dough into a slightly larger circle compared to the first one. Fit this dough into a 9 inch baking pan, with the edges hanging out.

Drain the artichokes, spinach, olives and the red pepper strips using paper towels and set aside.

Sauté the fresh mushrooms in a pan for about 8 minutes and drain off the excess liquid.

Now, layer half the mushrooms, salami and olives on the dough in the pan and top with half the cheese. Also layer with half the pepper strips, spinach and artichokes and repeat the layering ending with the cheese.

Combine the egg with water and lightly brush over the pastry edges. Cover with the remaining dough and fold the overhanging edges, pressing and crimping well to seal. Brush the top with the egg-water mixture.

Bake for about half an hour then remove from oven and immediately cover using aluminum foil, to prevent further browning.

Return to oven and bake for 15 more minutes. Place on a wire rack to cool off slightly then cut into wedges and serve.

Enjoy!

Quinoa veggie breakfast salad

Ingredients

3 ½ cups quinoa, cooked

1 ½ cups fresh/ frozen peas

4 cups red beans, cooked

½ yellow onion, diced

½ red/ orange bell peppers

½ cucumber, peeled then diced

1 ½ tbsp. extra virgin olive oil

1 ½ tbsp. extra virgin flax oil

2 tbsp. aged balsamic vinegar

Sea salt and freshly ground pepper

Directions

Soak all your grains for a minimum of six hours before cooking to neutralize the antinutrients found in grains.

Combine the cooked quinoa, veggies and beans in a large mixing bowl and toss well to combine evenly.

In a small bowl, mix the vinegar, oils, salt and pepper until well blended then pour over the salad.

Toss gently until evenly distributed the serve over a bed of lettuce. You can also let the salad marinate in your fridge overnight.

Enjoy!

Yummy Mexican Bowl

Ingredients

150g leftover ground beef

12 black olives, sliced into two

¼ yellow bell pepper, diced

½ avocado, diced

2 hardboiled eggs, mashed using a fork

1 tsp extra virgin olive oil

½ tsp cumin

¼ tsp onion powder

¼ tsp chili powder

1 tsp white wine vinegar

1 tomato, diced

1 tbsp. mayonnaise

Freshly squeezed juice of half a lime

Salt and pepper to taste

Coriander leaves for garnish

Directions

Combine the diced avocado with olive oil, vinegar, salt and pepper in a medium bowl and leave to marinade.

Meanwhile place a pan over medium to high heat and add the cooked minced meat, cumin, and half the tomato, chili and onion powders.

Cook for about a minute until the tomato softens, stirring occasionally.

Transfer the minced beef to a shallow bowl and arrange it around the sides and bottom of the bowl. Layer the remaining ingredients starting with the eggs, peppers, tomatoes, olives and finally the avocado.

Mix the cumin with the mayonnaise and drizzle over the top. Sprinkle the lime juice and garnish with coriander.

Enjoy!

Tasty Egg Mug

Ingredients

1 large egg

½ tomato, sliced

1/8 cup egg whites

3 fresh basil leaves

15g fresh mozzarella

1 tsp aged balsamic vinegar

Non-stick olive oil spray

Directions

Spray a mug with the olive oil cooking spray and add all the ingredients apart from the egg, balsamic and egg whites and pop in the microwave for half a minute.

Crack the egg and add to the mug together with the egg whites, stirring very gently with the other ingredients.

Pop in the microwave for 2 more minutes at the highest setting. Cook until well done then drizzle with the aged balsamic vinegar.

Let it stand for a minute or so and serve with crusty bread.

Yummy Greek Breakfast Sausage

Ingredients

450g minced lamb

450g minced pork

¼ cup ice water

4 cloves garlic, minced

¼ tsp cayenne pepper

1 tsp oregano

1 tsp fennel seed

1 tbsp. kosher salt

1 tsp ground coriander

Finely grated zest of 2 oranges

Directions

Combine the minced meats in a large bowl.

In a small separate bowl, combine all the spices and add them to the meat. Also add the ice water and use your hands to mix everything up.

Cover the bowl with plastic wrap and refrigerate for at least one hour up to overnight.

Divide the meat mixture into 16 portions and flatten to form rounded disks.

Heat some oil in a pan and fry the disks for about 3 minutes on each side or until well done then transfer to a plate lined with paper towels

Enjoy!

High Protein Blueberry Pancakes

Ingredients

2/3 cup blueberries

½ cup rolled oats, gluten free

½ tsp baking powder

1 tbsp. whole wheat flour

½ ripe banana

½ tsp vanilla extract

1 tsp vanilla almond milk

¼ cup pure maple syrup

1 pkt plain Greek yogurt

Directions

Combine all the ingredients apart from the maple syrup and blueberries. Let the mixture sit for about a minute in the bowl.

Use olive oil cooking spray to grease your pan or griddle and start cooking the pancakes for about 3 minutes on each side until golden.

Now, combine the blueberries and maple syrup in a small saucepan and cook until the berries soften and the mixture becomes syrupy.

Drizzle the blueberry sauce over the pancakes and serve immediately.

Light And Fluffy Eggy Muffins

Ingredients

Egg mixture:

4 eggs

1 tsp basil

½ tbsp. ground mustard

½ cup zero fay Greek yogurt

½ tsp cayenne pepper

The filling:

2 tbsp. extra virgin olive oil

3 slices bacon

2 jalapeno peppers, chopped

½ cup white onion, finely chopped

1/ tsp freshly ground black pepper

1 tsp kosher salt

1 tbsp. hot sauce, optional

Grated cheese for topping, optional

Directions

Start by baking the bacon. Set it aside and crumble once cooled.

Add the olive oil to a pan over medium to low heat and sauté the onions, jalapenos, black pepper and salt until the onions brown. Don't increase the heat as this will make the onions burn and not brown well.

Break the eggs into a large mixing bowl and combine with the yogurt and once it's well blended, add the ground mustard, basil, cayenne, baking powder, baking soda, crumbled bacon and the cooked veggies.

Spray the muffin tins with olive oil cooking spray and divide the mixture evenly.

Set your oven to 400F and bake for about 15 minutes. The muffins should puff up and turn golden at the tops.

If you are going to add cheese, sprinkle the tops and pop in the oven for a minute or so until melted.

Serve with hot sauce if so desired.

Enjoy!

Avocado, Bacon, Egg Sandwich

Ingredients

2 hardboiled eggs, Chopped

1 avocado, chopped

3 bacon slices, fried and crumbled

1 tbsp. Greek yogurt

2 green onions, sliced

¼ tsp garlic powder

¼ tsp Dijon mustard

Kosher salt and freshly ground pepper to taste

Directions

Combine all the ingredients in a large mixing bowl until well combined and spread on your favorite breakfast bread.

Enjoy!

Protein Rich Breakfast Smoothie

Ingredients

½ cup frozen blueberries

2 ripe bananas, sliced

5 frozen peach slices

1 tbsp. coconut oil

¼ tsp flaxseed

¼ tsp chia seeds

2 tbsp. Greek yogurt

4 cups fresh apple juice

Directions

Start by adding all the fruit to the blender followed by the seeds, coconut oil, and yogurt and apple juice.

Pulse until you achieve the desired consistency. Serve in a tall glass.

Enjoy!

Breakfast Poached Egg

Ingredients

4 eggs

4 bacon slices, fried and crumbled

4 tomato slices

1 cup extra virgin olive oil

1/3 cup pesto

2 slices garlic naan bread

5 small potatoes, washed and cubed

1 yellow onion, chopped

3 tbsp. garlic, chopped

½ cup fresh thyme

¼ cup fresh parsley

3 tbsp. white wine vinegar

2 slices cheddar cheese

Directions

Start by setting your oven to 250F and generously spread the pesto on the garlic naan slices and top with the cheddar slices.

Place in the oven for about 10 minutes until warmed through.

Add some of the olive oil to a large pan over medium to high heat and fry the onions, garlic and the cubed potatoes. Lower the heat and sauté until the potatoes turn golden.

Next bring a large pot of water to a boil. Ensure the water gets to a rolling boil then stir in the vinegar. Gently crack the eggs, one at a time into a bowl and lower to the boiling water.

For a great poached egg, swirl the water using a spoon before adding the eggs to ensure the egg whites are not separated from the yolk.

Do this for all the eggs.

Take out he naan slices from the oven and top with tomato slices, bacon and top with the poached egg. Season with sea salt and pepper, if desired.

Garnish with the fresh herbs and serve with the garlic potatoes and drizzle with extra olive oil.

Enjoy!

Energy Boosting Breakfast Smoothie

Ingredients

2 ripe bananas

1 tsp vanilla extract

2 tbsp. Greek yogurt

1 tsp natural honey

A good pinch cinnamon

2 ice cubes

Directions

Combine all the ingredients in your blender apart from the honey and pulse to desired consistency.

Serve on a tall glass and top with honey.

Enjoy!

Breakfast Cheesecake Smoothie

Ingredients

¼ cup blueberry reduced fat Greek yogurt

A handful baby spinach

1 cup frozen mixed berries

½ cup unsweetened almond milk

¾ cup water

30g low fat softened cream cheese

1 tbsp. ground flaxseed

1 tsp cinnamon

Natural honey to taste

Directions

Combine the baby spinach, water and mixed berries in your blender and pulse for 30 seconds. Add in the remaining ingredients to the blender and pulse for about 45 seconds or until you get the desired consistency.

Serve in a tall glass.

Enjoy!

Protein Power Breakfast

Ingredients

½ bunch grapes

1 orange

3 tbsp. oats or flaxseed or chia seeds, optional

3 tbsp. Greek yogurt

1 pear

Directions

Chop all the fruit into bite sized chunks and put them in a serving bowl.

Top with the Greek yogurt and oats, flaxseed or chia seeds, if desired.

Enjoy!

Baked Frittata With Pesto

Ingredients

8 eggs, beaten

¼ cup basil pesto

3 cloves garlic, minced

1 cup white onion, diced

330g bottled roasted red peppers, drained then sliced

2 handfuls baby arugula, torn

¼ tsp freshly ground black pepper

½ tsp kosher salt

1 tbsp. extra virgin olive oil

½ cup part skimmed mozzarella cheese

Directions

Set your oven to 350F and spray a large pie pan with olive oil cooking spray.

Add the olive oil to a large pan and place over medium heat and sauté the onions for about 5 minutes or until tender. Add in the garlic and sauté for one more minute until fragrant then remove from heat.

Combine the eggs, arugula, red peppers, pesto, and cheese, salt and pepper until well combined.

Bake in the prepared pie pan for about 40 minutes or until an inserted toothpick comes out very clean.

Remove from oven and let stand for 5 minutes before serving.

Enjoy!

Egg And Red Pepper Breakfast Bake

Ingredients

3 red bell peppers, cut into strips

6 eggs + 1 beaten egg for brushing

2 red onions, cut into thin wedges

6 tbsp. extra virgin olive oil

1 sheet puff pastry, thawed

4 tbsp. sour cream

1 tsp coriander

1 tsp cumin

A handful of cilantro, chopped

A handful of fresh parsley, chopped

2 fresh sprigs of thyme with the leaves removed

Freshly cracked pepper and salt to taste

Directions

Start by setting your oven to 400F.

Combine the onions, pepper, spices and thyme in a mixing bowl and drizzle with olive oil and toss well to combine.

Spread the veggies on a baking sheet and bake for half an hour, stirring 2-3 times so they roast evenly.

Sprinkle the roasted veggies with half of the fresh herbs then set aside.

Turn up your oven to 425F. Meanwhile, roll out the puff pastry until it forms a large square then divide it into 6 squares. Transfer the squares to 2 parchment papers.

Take a blunt knife and make a ¼ "frame around the square, careful not to go all the way through.

Prick the inside part of the square using the tines of a fork and refrigerate for half an hour.

Remove the pastry from the fridge and use a kitchen brush to lightly coat the pastry with the beaten egg.

Spread the insides of the 6 squares with the sour cream and top with the roasted veggies, leaving a shallow well at the center for the egg and leaving out a clear margin.

Place in the oven and bake for about 10 minutes until they start turning golden then remove from oven and crack an egg into each of the wells.

Return to the oven and bake for 10 more minutes. Remove from oven and season with cracked pepper, salt and the remaining herbs.

Drizzle with extra virgin olive oil and serve immediately. Enjoy!

Healthy Lunch Recipes

Chicken Greek Salad

Ingredients

330g cooked chicken, cubed

½ cup black olives, sliced

½ cup red onion, chopped

1/3 cup red wine vinegar

6 cups romaine lettuce, roughly torn

2 tomatoes, diced

2 tbsp. extra virgin olive oil

1 cucumber, peeled and chopped

½ cup crumbled feta cheese

1 tbsp. fresh dill, chopped or 1 tsp dried oregano

¼ tsp freshly ground pepper

1 tsp garlic powder

Kosher salt of flaky sea salt to taste

Directions

Whisk olive oil, red wine vinegar, dill/ oregano, salt, garlic powder and pepper in a large salad bowl.

Toss in the cubed chicken, lettuce, tomatoes, olives, cucumber, onion and feta cheese and mix well until evenly coated.

Note: if you don't have ready chicken, poach 450g chicken breast in a medium saucepan with salted water for about 15 minutes until cooked through. Set aside to cool then cut it in cubes.

Ketogenic Diet

Herbed Salmon Skewers

Ingredients

450g skinned center cut salmon fillet, cubed

450g cherry tomatoes

2 tsp. extra virgin olive oil

1 tsp freshly squeezed lemon juice

2 cloves garlic, minced

2 tsp. Fresh rosemary, minced

1 tsp lemon zest, freshly grated

¼ tsp freshly ground pepper

½ tsp kosher salt

Directions

Start by setting your grill to medium to high heat.

Mix the olive oil, rosemary, lemon juice and zest, garlic, salt and pepper in a mixing bowl then add the salmon cubes and gently toss to combine.

Make the skewers by alternating between the cherry tomatoes and the salmon.

Fold a paper towel and oil it with the olive oil then rub on the grill grate, holding the towel using tongs. It is not recommended to use cooking spray on a hot grill.

Grill the skewers for about 4 minutes, turning the skewers one until the fish is cooked through. Serve hot.

Enjoy!

Grilled Tuna With Relish

Ingredients

For the tuna:

750g tuna steak, divided into 6 portions

A good pinch freshly ground pepper

¼ tsp sea salt

1 tbsp. extra virgin olive oil

Lemon wedged, for garnishing

For the relish:

1/3 cup black olives, pitted and chopped

1 clove garlic, minced

½ cup fresh parsley, finely chopped

¼ cup celery, finely chopped

1 tbsp. freshly squeezed lemon juice

1 tsp extra virgin olive oil

A good pinch salt

Freshly ground pepper, to taste

½ tsp dried oregano

Directions

Start by preparing the relish by mixing the chopped olives, parsley, celery, olive oil, lemon juice, garlic, salt and pepper. Toss well to combine then aside.

For the tuna, rub olive oil on all sides of the steaks then season generously with the salt and pepper. Grill the tuna on medium to high heat for about 4 minutes on each side until well seared.

Serve immediately with the relish and garnish with lemon wedges.

Enjoy!

Tuna Antipasto Lunch Salad

Ingredients

330g water packed light tuna, drained then flaked

4 tsp. capers, rinsed

1 red bell pepper, finely chopped

4 tbsp. extra virgin olive oil

½ cup red onion, finely chopped

½ cup freshly squeezed lemon juice

300g canned chickpeas, rinsed and drained

8 cups arugula

½ cup fresh parsley, chopped

1 ½ tsp. fresh rosemary, finely chopped

¼ tsp sea salt

Freshly ground pepper, to taste

Directions

Combine the flaked tuna, chickpeas, capers, bell pepper, rosemary, onion, 2 tbsps. of olive oil and ¼ cup of the lemon juice in a salad bowl and season with pepper.

Combine the remaining olive oil, lemon juice and salt in a bowl then toss in the arugula until evenly coated. Divide the arugula on 4 serving plates and top with the tuna antipasto salad.

Enjoy!

Moroccan Veggie Soup

Ingredients

450g lamb stew meat, cubed

1 zucchini, peeled and diced

2 carrots, diced

1 yellow onion, finely diced

350g diced tomatoes

2 tbsp. extra virgin olive oil

2 tsp. turmeric powder

½ cup angel hair pasta, broken into 1 inch pieces

A pinch of saffron threads

2 stalks celery including the leaves, thinly sliced

6 cups reduced sodium, beef broth

8 sprigs fresh cilantro plus more for garnish

12 sprigs flat leaf parsley, plus more for garnish

½ tsp freshly ground pepper

½ tsp kosher salt

Directions

Add the oil to a Dutch oven set over medium to high heat then sauté the onion for about a minute then stir in the turmeric powder. Continue cooking until the onions become soft then add the meat and cook for 5-7 minutes.

Pour in the broth, turnips, and tomatoes together with the juice, celery, carrots and saffron. Use kitchen twine to tie the cilantro and parsley sprigs then add them to the cooking stew. Once the pot comes to a boil, reduce heat and simmer for about 50 minutes until the meat is nice and tender.

Add in the zucchini and cook for 10 minutes then add the pasta and cook for about 10 minutes, depending on the type of angel hair pasta you are using.

Discard the sprigs and season the stew with salt and pepper. Garnish with cilantro and parsley leaves.

Enjoy!

Yummy Rabbit Stew

Ingredients

1.3 kg fresh rabbit, divided into 6 large portions

¼ cup extra virgin olive oil

600g cherry tomatoes, cut in half

½ cup dry white wine

1 cup diced carrots

1 ½ cups peeled and diced potatoes

1 cup diced celery

¼ cup salt packed capers, rinsed

¼ cup red wine vinegar

¼ cup pine nuts

½ cup green olives, pitted and chopped

1 cup chopped red onion

¼ tsp freshly ground pepper

½ tsp sea salt

1 tbsp. natural honey

Directions

Season the rabbit with the salt and pepper on all sides.

Add 2 tbsps. of olive oil to a large wok over medium heat and brown the rabbit pieces for about4 4 minutes on each side. You can do this in batches if desired.

Once they are well browned, transfer to a shallow bowl. Pour the white wine into the wok and cook for 2 minutes until the wine reduces to a couple of tbsps. Pour this into the bowl containing the rabbit meat and cover to retain the heat.

Heat the remaining oil in the same wok and sauté the onion for about 3 minutes until translucent but not brown. Add the potatoes, carrots and celery and cook for 5 minutes, stirring frequently until they start becoming soft.

Add in the capers, olives, tomatoes and pine nuts and cook for 5 minutes until the tomatoes start getting mushy.

Return the rabbit meat together with all the juices to the wok, nestling the rabbit pieces into the veggies. Cover and simmer for 35 minutes until tender.

As the stew is cooking, whisk the honey and vinegar in a small pan and bring to a gentle boil then simmer for 5 minutes. Once the rabbit is almost cooked, stir in the honey reduction and cook for 10 minutes over medium heat.

Serve immediately.

Enjoy!

Grilled Tofu With Yummy Mediterranean Salad

Ingredients

400g water packed, extra firm tofu

¼ cup freshly squeezed lemon juice

3 cloves garlic, minced

1 tbsp. extra virgin olive oil

½ tsp sea salt

2 tsp. dried oregano

A good pinch freshly ground pepper, or to taste

see next recipe for yummy Mediterranean salad recipe

Directions

Start by setting your grill to medium to high heat.

Whisk the olive oil, lemon juice, oregano, garlic, salt and fresh pepper in a small mixing bowl. Set 2 tbsps. of this mixture aside, for basting the tofu.

Drain the tofu, rinse well the pat dry and cut it into 8 pieces then place in a shallow dish, preferably a glass one. Add the marinade to the dish and turn the tofu to coat well. Cover using cling wrap and refrigerate for half an hour or for 8 hours if you want deeper flavors.

Oil the grill grate using a folded paper towel that's been dipped in olive oil. Drain the tofu and grill for about 4 minutes on each side, basting with the reserved marinade.

Serve hot with the salad.

Enjoy!

Yummy Mediterranean Salad

Ingredients

1 cup seedless cucumber, diced

¼ cup Kalamata olives, pitted and roughly chopped

2 tomatoes, seeded and chopped

¼ cup chopped green onions

1 tbsp. white wine vinegar

2 tbsp. extra virgin olive oil

¼ cup fresh parsley, roughly chopped

¼ tsp flaky sea salt

Freshly ground pepper to taste

Directions

Combine all the ingredients in a salad bowl and toss well to combine.

Serve with the grilled tofu, within an hour of preparing.

Enjoy!

Tasty Mustard Crusted Salmon With Sour Cream

Ingredients

600g center cut salmon fillet, divided into 4 portions

2 tbsp. mustard, stone ground

¼ cup reduced fat sour cream

2 tsp freshly squeezed lemon juice

¼ tsp kosher salt

Freshly ground pepper, to taste

Lemon wedges for garnish

Directions

Start by setting your broiler to medium heat. Line a baking sheet with aluminum foil and lightly coat with olive oil cooking spray.

Arrange the salmon pieces on the baking sheet with the skin side down.

Season generously with salt and pepper.

Combine the mustard, sour cream and lemon juice in a bowl then pour over the salmon.

Broil for about 10 minutes when it is about 5 inches from the source of heat until it turns opaque.

Serve hot with lemon wedges.

Enjoy!

Simple Florentine Steaks

Ingredients

2 600g T-bone steaks

2 tsp. extra virgin olive oil

½ tsp freshly ground pepper

¾ tsp flaky sea salt

Directions

Make sure you remove the steaks from the fridge an hour or so before you start cooking.

Set your grill to high.

Rub the steak with pepper and grill for about 8 minutes on each side or until desired doneness is achieved.

Transfer the steaks to a cutting board, cover with aluminum foil and let rest for 5 minutes before cutting it up. Season with flaky sea salt and drizzle with olive oil.

Enjoy!

Strip Steak Served With Horse Radish Slaw

Ingredients

450g stripped steak, divided into 4 portions

3 cups shredded root veggies such as celeriac, carrots, beets or turnips.

¼ cup aged balsamic vinegar

1 ½ tbsp. Extra virgin olive oil

4 tbsps. Prepared horseradish

3 tbsp. fresh dill, chopped

¼ cup water

1 tbsp. reduced fat sour cream

¼ tsp freshly ground pepper

¾ tsp kosher salt

Directions

Mix the shredded root veggies with 2 tbsps. of dill, 2 tsps. olive oil and 1'2 a tsp. of kosher salt in a medium bowl. Toss well until evenly combined.

Rub the steaks with the remaining salt and pepper then set aside.

Add the 1 tbsp. of olive oil to a large pan over medium heat then sear the steaks for about 5 minutes on each side, adjusting the heat as required.

Turn off the heat and let the steaks rest on a paper toweled lined plate.

Add the vinegar, water and horseradish to the pan, scrapping up any browned bits. Drain any accumulated juice from the steaks into the pan and cook for about a minute. Drizzle half of this sauce over the veggies and toss well to coat evenly. Add sour cream and the remaining dill to the remaining sauce.

Serve the steaks in four plates and divide the slaw among the plates. Drizzle the sauce over the steaks and serve immediately.

Enjoy!

Brussel Sprouts Served With Bacon And Horseradish Cream

Ingredients

650g Brussel sprouts, trimmed and cut in half

2 tsp. prepared horse radish

4 strips bacon, cooked and crumbled

¼ cup reduced fat sour cream

A good pinch freshly ground pepper

¼ tsp. kosher salt

Directions

Place a steam basket into a large pot and add about one inch of water into the pot. Once it starts boiling, add the Brussel sprouts to the basket and steam for 8 minutes until tender.

Combine the bacon, horse radish, sour cream pepper and salt in a bowl then toss in the Brussel sprouts until evenly coated.

Enjoy!

Jumbo Shrimp Saganaki

Ingredients

900g jumbo shrimp, peeled, deveined with the tails left intact

1 bulb fennel, cored then finely chopped

½ cup Greek chardonnay

5 green onions, thinly sliced

1 tbsp. extra virgin olive oil

2 tbsp. freshly squeezed lemon juice

1 jalapeno, seeded and minced

½ cup crumbled feta cheese

¼ tsp kosher salt

Freshly ground pepper, to taste

Directions

Add 1 tbsp. of lemon juice to a bowl then toss in the shrimp until evenly coated then sprinkle with the salt.

Heat the olive oil in a saganaki pan then sauté the green onions, fennel and jalapeno over medium heat for about 5 minutes until they start turning golden. Stir in the wine and cook for a minute, stirring frequently.

Add the shrimp on the fennel mixture and cook covered for about 5 minutes until the shrimp are pink then turn off the heat.

Transfer the shrimp to a platter then add the cheese, remaining lemon juice and the pepper to the pan and cook for a minute, stirring constantly and you are ready to serve.

Enjoy!

Yummy Shrimp And Arugula Salad

Ingredients

450g raw shrimp, peeled and deveined

1 ½ cups cherry tomatoes, cut in half

1 ½ cups fresh corn kernels

2 cups whole grain herbed-garlic croutons

4 tbsp. extra virgin olive oil

12 cups arugula leaves

1 ½ tbsp. freshly squeezed lemon juice

1 ½ tbsp. aged balsamic

½ tsp kosher salt

2 tsp. grainy mustard

2 cups fresh basil, roughly torn

Freshly ground pepper, to taste

½ cup parmesan cheese, grated

Directions

Mix the tomatoes, arugula, corn and basil in a large mixing bowl. Separately whisk the lemon juice, 3 tbsps. of olive oil, mustard, vinegar and half the salt in a bowl.

Sprinkle the shrimp with the remaining kosher salt.

Heat 1 tbsp. of olive oil in a nonstick pan and cook the shrimp for 3 minutes or until they turn pink and opaque at the center.

Add the shrimp to the salad mixture together with the croutons then drizzle with the vinaigrette. Toss well until evenly coated then season with pepper and top with the grated cheese.

Enjoy!

Tasty Margarita Shrimp Summer Salad

Ingredients

For the salad:

450g shrimp (medium sized), peeled and deveined

2 cups endives, torn

2 ripe but firm avocadoes, cubed

1 orange, cut into segments

1 tbsp. extra virgin olive oil

¼ cup tequila

1 tsp fresh lime zest, grated

1 tbsp. freshly squeezed lime juice

2 tsp. fresh orange zest, grated

¼ cup red onion, thinly slivered

½ tsp. kosher salt4 cups romaine lettuce, torn

Lime wedges for garnish

For the dressing:

3 tbsp. freshly squeezed lime juice

1 tsp sugar

1 tsp chili powder

6 tbsp. reduced fat sour cream

2 tsp. jalapeno, seeded and minced

¼ tsp salt

Directions

For the dressing, whisk all the ingredients in a small bowl then set aside.

For the salad, toss the shrimp with the lime and orange zests, tequila and salt in a bowl cover using plastic wrap and refrigerate 10 minutes, tossing once or twice.

Cover the onion with ice cold water for 10 minutes to get rid of the sharpness.

Now toss the endives, lettuce and orange segments with the drained onion then drizzle with the salad dressing and toss well to combine. Serve the salad among four plates. Separately toss the cubed avocado with lime juice then add this to the salad.

Drain the shrimp and don't get rid of the marinade.

Add the olive oil to a large non-stick pan over medium heat and sauté the shrimp for about 3 minutes until pink. Divide the shrimp among the plates then add the retained marinade in the pan until it boils for about 3 minutes. Drizzle this over the shrimp and serve.

Enjoy!

Grilled Tofu With Salad Greens

Ingredients

For the tofu and salad greens:

700g water packed firm tofu, drained then rinsed well

2 tbsp. canola oil

2 tsp finely minced garlic

2 tbsp. reduced sodium soy sauce

10 ounces Asian salad greens

1 tbsp. black bean-garlic sauce

2 tbsp. natural honey

For the dressing:

½ cup fresh carrot juice

1 carrot, peeled and chopped

2 tbsp. rice vinegar

1 tbsp. fresh ginger, coarsely chopped

2 tbsp. extra virgin olive oil

2 tbsp. yellow miso

Directions

For the dressing, combine the ginger, carrot and carrot juice, vinegar, garlic, miso and oil in food processor or blender until you get a smooth consistency.

For the tofu, slice the tofu into 5 slices then dry using paper towels.

Combine the soy sauce, honey, garlic sauce, canola oil and garlic in a small bowl. Divide the marinade into two and spread half of it on a large baking dish then top with the tofu slices. Spread the remaining half of the marinade over the tofu until completely covered.

Set your grill on high and oil the grate using a folded paper towel that has been dipped in olive oil. Grill the tofu slices for 3 minutes on each side.

Toss the salad greens with the dressing and divide among 6 serving plates then top with the grilled tofu.

Enjoy!

Tofu Kebabs With Herbed Tomato And Onions

Ingredients

400g water packed extra firm tofu, drained and well rinsed

4 plum tomatoes, cut in quarters then seeded

1 tbsp. freshly squeezed lime juice

1 Vidalia onion, quartered then separated

1 tsp fresh ginger, minced

1 tbsp. reduced sodium soy sauce

2 jalapenos, seeded then diced

16 fresh mint leaves

¼ cup kecap manis (palm sugar sweetened soy sauce)

Directions

Divide the tofu into two, to form two large slices place a clean kitchen towel on a cutting board then place another clean kitchen towel on top of the tofu. Place a heavy weight on the towel such as a heavy bottomed pan then leave it to drain for about 20 minutes. Draining will help the tofu absorb all the flavors.

Now cut the tofu into pieces then set aside.

Set your grill on medium.

Meanwhile combine the ginger, lime juice and soy sauce in a large bowl then toss in the tofu and marinate for about 20 minutes.

As the tofu is marinating, stuff a mint leaf into each of the tomato quarters then thread the quarters with the onion, tofu and jalapenos in an alternating fashion in about 6 skewers.

Oil the grate using a folded paper towel dipped in olive oil and grill the skewers for about 7 minutes, turning the skewers 2 or 3 three times. Baste with the kecap manis and grill until the veggies start softening and the tofu browns for about 3 more minutes.

Enjoy!

Spicy Turkey With Avocado Relish

Ingredients

For the spicy turkey:

225g turkey cutlets

½ tsp 5-spice powder

2 tbsp. extra virgin olive oil

1 tbsp. chili powder

A good pinch kosher salt

For the avocado relish:

½ avocado, diced1 seedless grapefruit, cut into segments and discarding the membranes

1 small Vidalia onion, minced

1 tsp. red wine vinegar

1 tbsp. fresh cilantro, chopped

1 tsp natural honey

Directions

Combine the avocado, grapefruit segments, onion, honey, vinegar and cilantro and toss well to combine.

Next, combine all the spices for the turkey in a shallow bowl then dredge the cutlets in the spice mix.

Add the oil to a pan over medium heat and sear the turkey until cooked to desired doneness for about 3-5 minutes on each side.

Serve hot with the relish.

Enjoy!

Crab Bisque With Corn Relish

Ingredients

For the bisque:

330g crab meat

1 cup fresh corn

1 cup yellow pepper, diced

1 cup yellow onion, chopped 1 ½ cups potatoes, peeled and diced

1 cup dry sherry

2 cups almond milk

2 cups seafood broth

1 tbsp. extra virgin olive oil

¾ tsp sweet paprika

½ tsp kosher salt

For the relish:

1 cup fresh corn

1 avocado, finely cubed

1 tomato, seeded and finely chopped

1 tbsp. freshly squeezed lime juice

Freshly ground pepper, to taste

¼ tsp sea salt

Directions

For the relish, combine the corn, avocado, tomato, lime juice, pepper and salt in a bowl then toss well to combine then set aside.

Add the oil to a large sauce pot over medium heat and sauté the onion, corn and yellow pepper and cook for 5 minutes, stirring frequently.

Stir in the potato and sweet paprika for 2 minutes and pour in the sherry. Scrap up any browned bits and cook for 5 minutes. Pour in the broth and once it comes to a boil, lower the heat and simmer for 15 minutes or until the potatoes are very soft.

Puree this mixture in a food processor or blender, in two batches then return to the sauce pot. Stir in the crabmeat and the almond milk and season well with salt.

Cook for 5 minutes then serve with the relish.

Enjoy!

Tasty Seafood Salad

Ingredients

170g lump crab meat

4 medium-dry scallops, cut into quarters with the tough muscle removed

6 cherry tomatoes, cut in half

3 tbsp. white wine vinegar

1 small ruby red grapefruit, peeled and cut into segments with the membranes and seeds removed

1 avocado, diced

1 tsp Dijon mustard

2 tbsp. extra virgin olive oil

1 shallot, minced

3 cups romaine lettuce, shredded

¼ tsp freshly ground pepper

Flaky sea salt to taste

Directions

Add some water to a small saucepan and bring to a boil then add in the scallops and cook until opaque and firm for about a minute. Drain then rinse under cold water.

Whisk the mustard, shallot, salt, pepper and vinegar in a medium bowl then slowly whisk in the olive oil. Toss in the scallops and the crab in the dressing and toss well until evenly coated.

Combine the avocado, tomatoes, lettuce and the grapefruit then add the scallop mixture into the tomato mixture and toss well to combine.

Enjoy!

Simple Spring Salad

Ingredients

115g sardines, drained

2 hardboiled eggs

6 olives, pitted and cut in half

2 tbsp. extra virgin olive oil

½ bunch asparagus with the ends trimmed off

2 tbsp. red wine vinegar

1 clove garlic, crushed

10 cherry tomatoes, cut in half

¼ tsp dried tarragon

5 cups mixed salad greens

1 tsp whole grain mustard

A good pinch freshly ground pepper

Flaky sea salt to taste

Directions

Whisk the olive oil, mustard, vinegar, tarragon, pepper and sea salt in a bowl. Whisk in the garlic then set aside.

Boil a little water in a saucepan then add in the asparagus and cook for 3 minutes until crisp tender. Drain and place in an ice bath to retain the deep green color.

Peel the boiled eggs and slice them then set aside. Divide the mixed salad greens between two serving plates and top with the egg slices, tomatoes, sardines, asparagus and olives. Discard the garlic in the dressing then drizzle the dressing over the salads.

Enjoy!

Yummy Poached Halibut With Vinaigrette

Ingredients

For the halibut:

4 170g halibut steaks, skinned

1 tbsp. fresh chives, chopped

2 tbsp. canola oil

2 tsp. fresh dill, coarsely chopped with the sprigs for garnish

1 shallot, finely diced

1 tbsp. Dijon mustard

1 tbsp. fresh parsley, chopped

2 tbsp. freshly squeezed lemon juice

1 tbs. fresh tarragon, chopped

Sea salt and freshly ground pepper to taste

For the broth:

1 cup red wine vinegar

1 carrot, coarsely chopped

8 cups water

1 onion, cut into two

3 cloves garlic, roughly chopped with the peel on

1 tsp peppercorns

1 celery stalk, coarsely chopped

1 sprig fresh thyme

1 bay leaf

1 tbsp. kosher salt

Directions

Start by preparing the broth by combining all the ingredients in a large pot. Once it stats boiling, lower the heat and simmer for 30 minutes, uncovered then strain to another large pot and discard all the solids.

For the halibut, bring the both to a gentle simmer as you season the halibut with pepper and salt. Add the halibut to the broth and poach for 5-10 minutes, uncovered, until it turns opaque at the center.

Spoon 2 tbsps. of the broth into a bowl and combine it with lemon juice, sour cream and mustard. Slowly whisk in the oil then add the shallots.

Serve the halibut into 4 plates then stir in the herbs into the vinaigrette and spoon over the halibut and garnish with the dill sprigs.

Enjoy!

Roasted Cod With Olive Tapenade

Ingredients

450g cod fillet

1 cup cherry tomatoes, cut in half

1 tsp balsamic vinegar

3 tsp. extra virgin olive oil

1 tbsp. capers, well rinsed and chopped

¼ cup cured olives, chopped

1 tbsp. minced shallots

1 ½ tsp. fresh oregano, chopped

¼ tsp freshly ground pepper

Directions

Set your oven to 450F and coat a baking sheet with olive oil cooking spray.

Rub the cod fillet with 2 tsps. olive oil and generously sprinkle with pepper then place it on the prepared baking sheet. Roast for about 20 minutes until it flakes easily with a fork.

As the cod is roasting, heat the tsp. of oil in a small pan and sauté the shallots for 20 seconds until it starts softening. Stir in the tomatoes and cook for a minute or two until the tomatoes start softening. Add in the capers and the olives and cook for half a minute. Stir in the vinegar and the oregano then turn off the heat. Serve the tapenade over the cod.

Enjoy!

Fish Stew

Ingredients

600g swordfish, mahi-mahi or halibut steaks

6 canned plum tomatoes, coarsely chopped

¼ cup slat packed capers, rinsed

1 ½ cups yellow fleshed potatoes, peeled and thinly sliced

1 cup green olives

½ red onion

¼ cup extra virgin olive oil

2 celery stalks, diced

1 clove garlic, chopped

¼ cup flat leaf parsley, chopped

¼ tsp freshly ground pepper

A good pinch crushed red pepper

¼ tsp sea salt

Directions

Pat the fish steaks dry and season with salt and fresh pepper on both sides.

Mix the olive oil, celery, tomatoes, olives, onion, garlic, capers and red pepper in a pan and toss well to combine. Gently layer the thin potato slices until they completely cover the veggies.

Cover the pan and place over low heat. Cook for about 20 minutes and simmer gently, shaking the pan occasionally. Do not stir the veggies.

Add the fish on the potatoes, cover the pan and keep cooking for about 15 minutes until the fish turns opaque at the center. Garnish with parsley and serve.

Enjoy!

Mediterranean Kumquat Stew

Ingredients

2 cups kumquats, seeded and roughly chopped

900g skinned and boneless chicken thighs, cubed

4 cloves garlic, slivered

400ml low sodium vegetable broth

1 tbsp. minced ginger

2 yellow onions, thinly sliced

1 tbsp. extra virgin olive oil

1 ½ tbsp. natural honey

300g chickpeas, well rinsed

¾ tsp cinnamon powder

1 tsp coriander powder

½ tsp freshly ground pepper

1 tsp cumin powder

1/8 tsp ground cloves

½ tsp salt

Directions

Set your oven to 375 F.

Heat the olive oil in a Dutch oven and sauté the onions for 4 minutes until tender. Stir in the ginger and garlic and cook until fragrant, for about a minute.

Add in the chicken and cook for 8 minutes, stirring frequently then add all the spices and salt. Cook for about 30 seconds then stir in the chickpeas, kumquats and honey then bring to a gentle simmer.

Cover and transfer to the oven and bake for about an hour until the chicken is cooked through.

Serve hot.

Enjoy!

Tasty Appetizer and Dinner Recipes

Veggie Salad Kabobs

Ingredients

24 tooth picks

24 small grape tomatoes

3 English cucumbers, sliced and halved

24 Kalamata olives, pitted

2 tsps. honey

1 small clove garlic, finely chopped

2 tsps. fresh oregano, chopped

2 tsps. fresh dill weed, chopped

¼ tsp salt

¾ cup low fat plain Greek yoghurt

Directions

Mix yoghurt, oregano, dill, honey, garlic and salt in a bowl and set aside.

Thread an olive, a tomato, half a slice of cucumber on each tooth pick and serve with the dip.

Simple Salsa Recipe

Ingredients

1 cup zucchini, finely chopped

1 ½ cups tomatoes, seeded and chopped

½ cup roasted bell peppers, finely chopped

1 garlic clove, minced ☐ 1 ½tsp capers

1 tbsp. fresh flat leaf parsley, chopped

1 tbsp. fresh basil, chopped

2 tbsps. red onion, finely chopped

2 tsps. lemon juice

2 tsps. olive oil

A pinch of salt

A pinch of black pepper, freshly ground

Directions

Combine all ingredients in a bowl and serve immediately or refrigerate.

Enjoy!

Yummy Tapenade

Ingredients

1 cup Kalamata olives, pitted

Juice of 1 lemon

2 tbsps. olive oil

5 cloves garlic

¼ cup parsley, chopped

1 tbsp. capers

½ tsp all spice

Directions

Place all the ingredients in a food processor and process until all ingredients combine well.

Serve in 8 small bowls.

Enjoy!

Mango Salsa

Ingredients

1 cup cucumber, chopped

2 cups mango, diced

½ cup cilantro, minced

2 tbsps. fresh lime juice

1 tbsp. scallions, minced

¼ tsp chipotle powder

¼ tsp sea salt

Directions

Mix together all ingredients in a bowl and serve or refrigerate. Enjoy!

Mediterranean Layered Dip

Ingredients

½ cup feta cheese, crumbled

½ a liter lemon yoghurt

1 tsp lemon juice, fresh

1 cup plain hummus

½ cup English cucumber, finely chopped

2 tbsps. green onions, chopped

½ cup Kalamata olives, pitted and chopped

½ cup tomatoes, seeded and chopped

1 tbsp. fresh parsley, chopped

Salt to taste

Directions

Mix cheese, yoghurt, lemon juice and salt in a small bowl.

Line up 8 glasses and layer 2 tbsps. Hummus, 1 tsp tomato, 1 tbsp. of yoghurt mixture, 1 tbsp. of cucumber, I tbsp. olives and 1 tsp green onions.

Top with the remaining ingredients.

Enjoy!

Classic Mediterranno Chicken

Ingredients

6 chicken breasts, skinned and deboned

3 cups tomatoes, chopped

½ cup onion, chopped

3 cloves garlic, pressed

½ cup calamite olives

½ cup white wine

¼ cup fresh parsley, chopped

2 tsp. extra virgin olive oil

2 tsps. fresh thyme, chopped

Salt and all spice to taste

Directions

Heat the oil and 3 tbsps. white wine in a skillet over medium heat. Add the chicken and cook for about 6 minutes on each side until golden. Remove the chicken and put it on a plate.

Add garlic and onions in the skillet and sauté for about 3 minutes and add the tomatoes. Let them cook for five minutes then lower the heat and add the remaining white wine and simmer for 10 minutes. Add the thyme and simmer for a further 5 minutes.

Return the chicken to the skillet and cook on low heat until the chicken is well done. Add olives and parsley and cook for 1 more minute. Add the salt and pepper and serve.

Enjoy!

Classic Penne And Chicken

Ingredients

1 packet penne pasta

750g chicken breasts, deboned and skinned, cut in halves

1 can artichoke hearts, soaked in water, chopped

½ cup feta cheese, crumbled

1 tomato, chopped

½ cup red onion, chopped

2 cloves garlic, pressed

3 tbsps. fresh parsley, chopped

1 ½ tbsps. butter or 3 tbsp. extra virgin olive oil

2 tbsps. lemon juice

Salt and black pepper, freshly ground to taste

1 tsps. oregano, dried

Directions

Cook the penne pasta until al Dante in a large saucepan with salted boiling water.

Melt butter or heat olive oil in a large skillet over medium heat and add the onions and garlic. Cook these for 2 minutes and add the chicken. Stir occasionally until the chicken is golden brown for about 6 minutes.

Drain the artichoke hearts and add them to the skillet together with the cheese, lemon juice, tomatoes, oregano and drained pasta. Reduce the heat to medium low and cook for 3 minutes.

Add the salt and pepper to taste and serve warm.

Enjoy!

Hearty Protein Rich Stew

Ingredients

2 cups zucchini, cubed

500g beef (chuck), cubed

2 cups eggplant, cubed

1 can tomato sauce

1 packet frozen okra, thawed

1 butternut squash, peeled, seeded and diced

1 cup onion, chopped

2 tbsp. extra virgin olive oil

1 clove garlic, chopped

½ cup vegetable broth

1 carrot, thinly sliced

1 tomato, chopped

1/3 cup raisins

¼ tsp paprika

½ tsp Cumin, ground

½ tsp turmeric, ground

¼ tsp cinnamon, ground

¼ tsp red pepper, crushed

Directions

Combine everything in a slow cooker, cover and cook for 10 hours or until vegetables are tender.

Enjoy!

Yummy Herbed Chicken

Ingredients

8 chicken breasts, skinned, deboned and halved

1 medium red bell pepper, diced

1 small onion, thinly sliced

4 cloves garlic, pressed

¼ cup dry vermouth

¼ cup fresh parsley, chopped

1 ½ tbsps. corn starch

¼ tsp coarsely ground pepper

½ tsp dried oregano

2 tsps. dried rosemary

2 tbsps. cold water

Salt to taste

Directions

Combine onion, garlic, bell pepper, rosemary and oregano in a slow cooker. Crumble the sausages over the mixture, casings removed. Arrange the chicken in a single layer over the sausage and sprinkle with pepper. Add the vermouth and slow cook for 7 hours.

Move the chicken to a warm and deep platter and cover.

Mix the corn starch with the water in a small bowl and add this to the liquid in the slow cooker. Increase the heat and cover. Cook for about 10 minutes and season with salt. Pour the soup over the chicken and garnish with parsley.

Enjoy!

Tasty Spanish Cod

Ingredients

6 cod fillets

½ cup green olives, chopped

15 cherry tomatoes, halved

¼ cup onion, finely chopped

1 cup tomato sauce

1 tbsp. butter

2 tbsps. garlic, chopped

1 tbsp. extra virgin olive oil

1 dash cayenne pepper

1 dash black pepper

1 dash paprika

¼ cup deli marinated Italian vegetable salad, drained and chopped

Directions

Place a large skillet over medium heat and add the olive oil and butter. Add the onion and garlic and cook until garlic starts browning. Add the tomato sauce and tomatoes and let them simmer.

Stir in the marinated veggies, olives and spices. Cook the fillet in the sauce for 8 minutes in medium heat.

Serve immediately.

Enjoy!

Ketogenic Diet

Simple Grilled Tuna

Ingredients

4 tuna steaks, 1 inch thick

Fresh juice of 1 lime

3 tbsps. extra virgin oil

Salt and black pepper, freshly ground to taste

½ cup hickory wood chips, soaked

Directions

Place tuna and the olive oil in a zip lock plastic bag, seal and refrigerate for an hour.

Prepare a charcoal or gas grill. When using a coal grill, scatter a handful of hickory wood chips when the coals are hot for added flavor.

Lightly grease the grill grate and season the tuna with pepper and salt and cook on the grill for about 6 minutes turning only once.

Transfer to a plate and drizzle the lime juice and serve immediately.

Enjoy!

Roasted Lamb Chops

Ingredients

8 lamb loin chops, fat trimmed off

1 tbsp. dried oregano

1 tbsp. garlic, minced

2 tbsps. lemon juice, fresh

¼ tsp black pepper, freshly ground

½ tsp salt

Olive oil Cooking spray

Directions

Preheat your broiler

In a small bowl, combine all the spices, herbs and lemon juice and rub this mixture on both sides of the lamb chops.

Spray the broiler pan with the cooking spray and broil the lamb chops for 4 minutes on each side or depending on how done you want your chops.

Cover the cooked lamb chops in foil and let them rest for 5 minutes and you are ready to serve.

Enjoy!

Lemony Chicken Soup

Ingredients

1 whole chicken, well cleaned

1/3 cup uncooked white rice

salt and freshly ground black pepper to taste

2 eggs, beaten

1¼ lemons, juiced

Directions

Place the chicken in a pot large enough to hold it and to get around, but not too much space or your broth will end up being watery. Fill the pot with about 1 inch of water. Cover and bring to a boil then lower the heat and simmer for 45 minutes to 1 hour, skimming the fat from the top, as it accumulates.

When the chicken is cooked, the meat should pull easily from the bones. Transfer the cooked chicken to a large bowl and let cool.

Add the rice to the broth and season with salt and pepper. Simmer for 20 minutes or until rice is soft.

Beat the eggs with the lemon juice in a bowl. While beating the eggs, slowly trickle in the hot soup and stir well, this will temper the eggs and ensure they do not curdle

Gently add the egg mixture to the hot soup, stirring vigorously. The result should be a creamy and cloudy soup. You can season with additional salt, pepper or lemon juice at this point.

Add pieces of chicken in the soup and serve.

Ketogenic Diet

Enjoy!

Winter's Veggie Soup

Ingredients

1 cup chopped baby carrots

1 baking potato, cut into cubes

1/2 small sweet onion, chopped

1 stalk celery, chopped

500g beef, soft cut

1/4 small head cabbage, chopped

400g can diced tomatoes

1 cup cut fresh green beans (1/2 inch pieces)

600ml chicken broth

400ml can vegetable stock

1 cup water

3/4 tsp. dried basil

1/2 pinch rubbed sage

1/2 pinch dried thyme leaves

salt to taste

Directions

Combine carrots, potato, onions, celery, beef, cabbage, tomatoes, green beans, chicken broth, vegetable broth, water, basil, sage, thyme and salt in a large saucepan;

Bring to a boil then reduce heat and cover. Simmer until the vegetables are soft and the beef tender, for about 90 minutes.

Serve hot!

Enjoy!

Crab Chowder Soup

Ingredients

1/2 medium onion, chopped

2 tbsps. butter or extra virgin olive oil

1/6 cup all-purpose flour

1 ½ cups almond milk

2 bacon strips, cooked and crumbled

450g crabmeat, drained

1 medium potato, diced

1/2 small green pepper, chopped

1/2 celery rib, chopped

350g whole kernel corn, drained

1/2 cup half-and-half cream

1 bay leaf

1/2 tbsp. chopped fresh parsley

1/2 tsp. salt

1/8 tsp. ground nutmeg

1/8 tsp. white pepper

Directions

In a large pot sauté onions in butter or olive oil until tender. Next, stir in the flour until well combined Cook and stir until the mixture thickens and becomes bubbly.

Gradually pour in the almond milk stirring constantly until thick. Add the remaining ingredients. Cover and simmer until the vegetables are soft, about 35-40 minutes.

Remove bay leaf before serving into individual bowls.

Enjoy!

Arroz Con Pollo

Ingredients

1 cup water

3/4 cup uncooked long-grain rice (not quick cooking)

1/2 tsp. paprika

2 tbsp. extra virgin olive oil

1/2 tsp. black pepper

1 (10 3/4 ounce) can cream of mushroom soup

4 boneless skinless chicken breast halves/ drumsticks/ thighs

Directions

Preheat oven to 375 F.

Combine soup, water, rice and 1/4 tsp. each paprika and pepper in a shallow ungreased pan.

Place the chicken on top and sprinkle with paprika and pepper remains and drizzle with olive oil.

Cover and cook in oven until bubbly and chicken shows no signs of pink in the center – for about 45 minutes.

Enjoy!

A Tasty Twist On The Classic Meatloaf

Ingredients

350g ground beef

1 egg, divided

1/2 onion, chopped

1/2 cup milk

1/2 cup dried bread crumbs

salt and pepper to taste

1 tbsp. brown sugar

1 tbsp. prepared mustard

2 tbsps. and 2 tsps. ketchup

Directions

Preheat oven to 350 F

In a large bowl, combine the meat, half the egg (refrigerate the remaining half), onions, milk and bread or cracker crumbs. Season with salt and pepper and lightly greased 5x9 inch loaf pan, or a pan with the shape of a loaf and lightly greased 9x13 inch baking dish in one.

In a small bowl, brown sugar, mustard and ketchup. Mix well and pour over the meatloaf.

Bake at 350 F for 1 hour.

Enjoy!

Hearty Pot Roast

Ingredients

2 tsps. olive oil

1.8kg boneless chuck roast, trimmed

1 tbsp. kosher salt

1 tbsp. cracked black pepper

2 cups coarsely chopped onion

2 cups low-salt beef broth

1/4 cup ketchup

2 tbsps. Worcestershire sauce

1 cup chopped plum tomato

600g pounds small red potatoes

450g carrots, peeled and cut into 1-inch pieces

2 tbsps. fresh lemon juice

Chopped fresh parsley (optional)

Directions

Preheat oven to 400 F.

Add olive oil to a large saucepan over medium heat and meanwhile sprinkle the roast with salt and pepper. Add the roast into the pan, brown on all sides (about 8 minutes). Remove from pan and add onion to skillet; cook 8 minutes or until golden brown. Return to the pan and combine broth, tomato sauce and Worcestershire sauce; Pour over roast. Add tomatoes and bring to a boil.

Cover and bake at 400 F for 2 1/2 hours or until tender. Add the potatoes and carrots; Cover and cook 30 minutes or until vegetables are tender. Add the lemon juice and garnish with parsley, if desired.

Serve with mashed potatoes.

Enjoy!

Tasty Liver With Caramelized Onions

Ingredients

450g sliced beef liver

3/4 cup milk, for soaking

2 tbsps. butter or olive oil, divided

1 large Vidalia onions, sliced into rings

1 cup all-purpose flour, or as needed

A handful fried bacon bits, optional

salt and pepper to taste

Directions

Gently rinse the liver slices under cold water, and place them in a medium bowl. Pour in enough milk to cover the liver and let stand while preparing onions. This step is VERY important as it takes out the bitterness out of the liver

Melt 2 tbsps. of butter or olive oil in a large skillet over medium heat. Separate onion rings, and sauté them in butter until soft. Remove onions, and melt remaining butter in the skillet. Season the flour with salt and pepper, and put it in a shallow dish or on a plate. Drain milk from liver, and coat slices in the flour mixture.

When the butter has melted, turn the heat up to medium-high, and place the coated liver slices in the pan. Cook until nice and brown on the bottom. Turn, and cook on the other side until browned. Add onions, and reduce heat to medium. Cook a bit longer to taste. Enjoy!

Spicy Mahi-Mahi

Ingredients

1 3/4 tsps. ground cumin

1/2 tsp. garlic powder

1/2 tsp. dried oregano

1/4 tsp. ground ginger

1/4 tsp. smoked paprika

1/4 tsp. kosher salt

1/4 tsp. ground black pepper

1/8 tsp. ground red pepper

1 tbsp. olive oil

2 Mahi Mahi fillets

Grilling Spray

225g Stewed Tomatoes, drained, chopped

1/2 medium mango, peeled, chopped

1/2 jalapeno pepper, seeded, chopped

1/4 cup chopped red onion

1 tbsp. chopped fresh cilantro

1/2 tsp. ground cumin

1/2 tsp. minced garlic

1/2 lime, juiced

Directions

Mix ¾ tsp. cumin, garlic powder, dried oregano, ground ginger, smoked paprika, salt and red and black pepper in a small bowl. Add in olive oil to make a spicy paste; divide mixture in half and set one portion aside.

Rub half of the spice mix on the fish fillets then put aside. Coat the grill or barbecue with the grill spray and set to high heat; when hot, add the fish and cook for 3-4 minutes per side, turning once.

Drain tomatoes and combine with mango, chili, red onion, cilantro, 1 tsp. cumin, and garlic and lemon juice in a medium bowl; put aside.

Remove grilled fish as soon as it easily flakes when pierced with a fork. Brush the remaining fish remaining spice rub and serve with cooked pasta and mango salsa.

Enjoy!

Classic Meat Balls

Ingredients

600g ground beef

2 small eggs

1 ¼ slices toast, crumbled

1 medium onion, very finely minced

1/2fresh tomato

1/2 tbsp. dried mint, crushed

1 ¼ tbsps. Romano cheese, grated

2 tbsps. water

1/2 lemon, juice of

A dash cinnamon

1/2 to taste salt and pepper, to taste

1/2 to taste flour

canola oil, for frying

Directions

Skin the tomato and crush in blender.

Add to meat, mixing well.

Add remainder of ingredients except the flour and oil; mix lightly but thoroughly.

Form into small (about the diameter of a quarter) balls and roll lightly in flour.

Ketogenic Diet

Fry in hot oil until evenly browned; drain on paper toweling.

Serve hot as an appetizer.

Enjoy!

Mediterranean Fasolakia

Ingredients

1/4 cup extra virgin olive oil

1 cup onion

225g green beans

1/4 tsp. pepper

225g tomato paste

1 ½ cups parsley

3 potatoes, cut in cubes

2 tsps. salt

28g carrot

Directions

Heat oil in heavy large nonstick skillet over medium-high heat.

Add onion and sauté for 5 minutes.

Add green beans and cayenne pepper and sauté until onion is translucent, about 3 minutes.

Add potatoes and parsley.

Pour tomato paste over vegetables.

Bring to boil.

Reduce heat.

Cover and simmer until potatoes are tender, stirring frequently, about 45 minutes.

Season with salt and pepper.

Remove from heat.

Serve warm or at room temperature.

Enjoy!

Healthy Veggie Dish

Ingredients

1 small zucchini, halved lengthwise, then sliced into half-moons

1 medium tomatoes, large dice

1/2 tbsp. extra-virgin olive oil

1/2 tbsp. butter

1 ½ tbsp. parmesan cheese, grated

1/4 tsp. basil

1/4 tsp. pepper

Directions

In a large skillet sauté the zucchini and tomatoes in hot oil and butter for 5 minutes.

Add the Parmesan, pepper and basil.

Stir to coat well.

Serve warm. Enjoy!

Alfredo Chicken

Ingredients

90g dry fettuccine pasta

150g cream cheese

5 tbsps. extra virgin olive oil

1/4 cup almond milk

1/4 tsp. garlic powder

salt and pepper to taste

1 skinless, boneless chicken breast halves - cooked and cubed

1 cup chopped fresh broccoli

1 small zucchini, julienned

1/4 cup chopped red bell pepper

Directions

Bring a large pot of lightly salted water to a boil. Add in pasta and cook for 8-10 minutes, or cook until al dente; Drain.

While the pasta is cooking, melt the cream cheese and olive oil in a saucepan over low heat. Stir until smooth. Add milk and season with garlic powder, salt and pepper. Simmer for 3 minutes or until thickened, stirring constantly.

Take chicken, broccoli, zucchini and peppers. Cook 3 minutes at medium heat, then reduce the heat and simmer 5 minutes or until vegetables are tender. Serve over noodles. Enjoy!

Pork Served With Sauerkraut

Ingredients

900g pork loin roast

1/4 tsp. caraway seeds

1/4 tsp. black pepper

1/2 small baking apple, peeled, cored and diced very small or 1/3 cup apple sauce

450g sauerkraut, undrained

1/8 cup packed brown sugar

2 tbsps. butter, melted

1/2 to taste salt, if needed, to taste

Directions

Place the pork in a clay pot. Sprinkle with cumin and black pepper.

Put the diced apples (or applesauce) on top of the pork.

Pour the juice and sauerkraut.

Evenly sprinkle brown sugar on top of sauerkraut.

Sprinkle the tops with the melted butter.

Cook for about 8 hours or until pork reaches an internal temperature of at least 160 degrees Celsius

Stir in sauerkraut around a bit before serving. Enjoy!

Turnip Rice with Fried Pork

Ingredients:

Pork:

450g pork shoulder

2 cloves garlic, minced

1 tsp tomato paste

1 tsp hoisin sauce

½ tbsp. low sodium soy sauce

½ tsp sweet paprika

¼ tsp sesame oil

½ tbsp. sherry

¼ tsp five spice powder

½ tbsp. raw honey

½ tbsp. extra virgin olive oil

½ tbsp. hot water

A good pinch salt and white pepper

Turnip rice:

3 turnips

1 white onion

2 eggs

1 tbsp. low sodium soy sauce

1 tsp sesame oil

½ tbsp. extra virgin olive oil

4 scallions

Directions

Whisk together all the ingredients of the pork marinade in a mixing bowl and set aside 2 tablespoons. Cut the pork into about 3" pieces and place in a zip lock bag or airtight container, then pour in the marinade. Shake well and chill in the fridge for at least 4 hours or preferably overnight.

Meanwhile, chop the scallions and the white onion and place in the fridge.

Once the pork is ready, pre-heat the oven to 455F and line your baking tray with kitchen foil, then place a rack on top.

Place the marinated pork on the rack for about 25 minutes and baste it using the juices that have poured on the baking tray plus the remaining marinade. Bake for 20 more minutes, then broil the pork for 2 minutes to make it crisp on the outside but don't let it burn.

Remove the pork from the oven and brush it with the reserved 2 tablespoons of marinade and let it stand for 10 minutes before cutting it up.

Now peel the turnips and spiralize into noodles. Place the noodles in a food processor and pulse until it forms turnip rice then set aside.

Place a medium skillet on medium heat, coat with cooking spray then scramble the eggs and transfer them to a plate.

Wipe the skillet and pour in the olive oil and place on medium heat. Sauté the onions for 3 minutes then stir in the pork and turnip rice. Allow to cook for 5 minutes till the turnip becomes soft. Stir in the sesame oil, soy sauce, scrambled eggs, scallions and white pepper and cook for 2 minutes until they are heated through.

Enjoy!

Celery Root with Lamb Ragu

Ingredients:

1 celery root, spiralized

400g lean minced lamb

½ carrot, finely chopped

½ yellow onion, finely chopped

1 clove garlic, minced

½ celery stalk, finely chopped

250 g crushed tomatoes

½ tsp fresh thyme, chopped

½ tsp fresh rosemary, chopped

½ tbsp. olive oil

½ tbsp. tomato paste

¼ tsp red pepper flakes

1tbsp fresh mint, chopped

½ cup homemade chicken broth

1 tsp ground cumin

Kosher salt and freshly ground pepper to taste

Directions:

Combine the minced lamb, rosemary, cumin, thyme, garlic, salt and pepper in a pot and place over medium heat. Use a wooden spoon to loosen the lumps and cook until it is well browned. Stir in the celery, carrot, onion and red pepper flakes and cook for about 5 minutes until the vegetables become soft.

Add the tomatoes and stir in the tomato paste and the stock. Once the sauce starts boiling, lower the heat and bring to a gentle simmer for 20 minutes.

Meanwhile, add the olive oil in a large skillet and place over medium heat, then sauté the celery root noodles. Cover and cook for up to 10 minutes until the noodles are al dente, stirring occasionally. Add a bit of the broth if the noodles start sticking to the bottom.

Divide the cooked noodles into serving bowls together with the lamb ragu and garnish with fresh mint. Enjoy!

Tasty Pork Tenderloin

Ingredients

1 ½ kg pork tenderloin

2 tbsp. herbs de providence

2 tbsp. coconut oil

½ cup aged balsamic vinegar

1 tbsp. garlic powder

1 bell pepper, sliced

1 onion, sliced

Freshly ground pepper

Sea salt

Directions

Start by preheating your oven to 400 F and combine all the spices in a small bowl.

Heat the coconut oil in an oven proof skillet over high heat.

Rub all sides of the pork with the spice mix and sear in shimmering hot oil until it browns on all sides. This step is very important as it will help lock in the moisture.

Remove from pan and toss in the onions and bell pepper. Sprinkle with salt and pepper and toss the pork back in.

Put the skillet in the oven and bake for 20 minutes. Do not cover the skillet. Meanwhile, heat the balsamic vinegar over low heat and let simmer until it reduces by half then let cool.

Remove from oven and let sit for 10 minutes before slicing it up then drizzle with the balsamic glaze. Enjoy!

Chicken Veggie Casserole

Ingredients

8 chicken legs, deboned and cut into cubes

1 sweet potato, peeled and cut into cubes

2 cups Brussel sprouts

1 broccoli head

1 can coconut milk, full fat

1 clove garlic, minced

1 pearl onion, diced

2tbsp coconut oil

1 tbsp. Italian seasoning, plus 1 teaspoon more

Sea salt, to taste

Freshly ground pepper, to taste

Directions

Start by preheating your oven to 400 F and line a baking sheet with parchment paper.

Toss the potato cubes with a tablespoon of the Italian seasoning and a tablespoon of coconut oil in a medium bowl then place them on the prepared baking sheet. Bake for 25 minutes until tender.

Meanwhile, heat the remaining oil in a skillet over medium heat and toss in the onions and sauté until soft. Add the garlic and cook until fragrant for about 2 minutes. Now toss in the chicken and cook for 10 minutes until juices run clear, stirring every once in a while.

Cut off the broccoli stem and cut the Brussel sprouts in half. Add the two veggies to the chicken and cook for 2 more minutes then turn off the heat.

Sauce:

Combine the roasted potatoes, coconut milk and remaining seasoning in your food processor or blender and pulse until smooth.

Lightly grease a baking dish and scoop in the chicken mix, including any juices. Gently pour in the sauce to cover the chicken mix evenly. Place the baking dish in the oven and bake for half an hour.

Remove from oven and let sit for 8-10 minutes then serve. Yum!

Crispy, Spicy, Yummy Italian Chicken Thighs

Ingredients

500g chicken thighs

1 tsp red pepper flakes

1 tsp sweet paprika

1 tsp freshly ground black pepper

1 tsp dried oregano

1 tsp curry powder

1 tbsp. garlic powder

1-2 tbsp. coconut oil

Directions

Start by preheating your oven to 400 F and preparing a baking sheet by lining it with parchment paper.

Combine all the spices in a small bowl then set aside.

Now arrange the thighs on your prepared baking sheet with the skin side down (remember to first pat the skin dry with kitchen towels).

Sprinkle the upper side of the chicken thighs with half the seasoning mix, flip them over and sprinkle the lower side with the remaining seasoning mix.

Bake for about 40 minutes until the chicken thighs are cooked through and the skin is crisp. To make the skin crispier, turn on your broiler to high and broil the chicken thighs for 5 minutes.

Enjoy!

Tropical Island Salmon

Ingredients

Salmon:

4 salmon fillets with the skin on, about 6oz each

Freshly ground pepper

Flaky Maldon sea salt

Coconut oil

Salsa:

1 huge mango, peeled and cubed

2 tsp fresh coriander, finely chopped

¾ tsp Serrano chili, seeded and minced

½ red bell pepper, diced

½ red onion, finely chopped

2 tbsp. freshly squeezed lime juice

Sea salt

Directions

Salmon:

Start by preheating your oven to 350 F and set your baking rack at the center position.

Gently rub the fillets with salt and pepper and set aside.

Place an oven proof pan over medium heat and add about 2 tablespoons of coconut oil. Once the oil is shimmering hot, gently place the salmon on the pan with the skin side up and cook for 3 minutes then flip over and cook for a minute. Turn off the heat and place the pan in the oven and bake for 10 minutes until cooked through.

Meanwhile, combine all the salsa ingredients and chill in the fridge.

Once the salmon is ready, serve with the salsa and enjoy!

Tip: the salsa tastes even better when you prepare it at least 6 hours in advance so the flavors have time to meld.

Crowd Pleaser Slow Cooker Chili

Ingredients

2kg coarsely ground beef/ pork

2 cans diced tomatoes

6 jalapenos, deseeded and chopped

2 bell peppers, diced

4 hot yellow peppers, deseeded and chopped

2 poblanos, deseeded and chopped

½ tbsp. cacao powder

2 tbsp. ancho Chile powder

2 tbsp. cumin

2 tbsp. garlic powder

2 tbsp. ground coriander

2 tbsp. dried oregano

¼ cup low sodium beef broth, preferably homemade

2 tbsp. arrow root powder

Directions

Start by browning your beef in a skillet, in batches before putting it in your slow cooker, draining any excess fat in the process. Once all the beef is in your slow cooker, heat a bit of oil in the same skillet you used to brown the beef and sauté the veggies until tender. Stir in all the seasonings and continue cooking until the skillet dries up.

Drain the tomatoes and add them to the skillet. Stir well then transfer all the contents of the skillet to your slow cooker. Do not stir just layer the veggies on top then pour in the broth. Cover the cooker and turn it on and cook for 5-8 hours on low.

When you have about an hour to the end of cook time, mix the arrow root powder with a little water then pour it in the slow cooker together with the cacao powder, cover and continue cooking.

Taste and adjust seasonings as desired and you are ready to indulge. Enjoy!

Classic Salisbury Steak

Ingredients

2 (10.5 ounce) cans condensed French onion soup

1.2 kg ground beef

1 cup dry brown bread crumbs

2 eggs

1/2 teaspoon salt

1/4 teaspoon ground black pepper

2 tablespoons all-purpose flour

1/2 cup organic ketchup

1/2 cup water

2 tablespoons Worcestershire sauce

1 teaspoon mustard powder

Directions

In a large bowl, mix 1/3 cup condensed French onion soup with ground beef, bread crumbs, egg, salt and black pepper. Design 6 oval patties.

In a large skillet over medium heat, brown both sides of the patties. Drain off any excess fat.

In a small bowl, combine the flour and the rest of the soup until smooth. Mix the tomato sauce, water, Worcestershire sauce and mustard.

Pour over the meat in the pan. Cover and simmer for 20 minutes, stirring occasionally. Serve hot with mashed potatoes. Enjoy!

Zoodles with Tasty Lentil Marinara

Ingredients:

6 zucchini, spiralized into noodles

1 cup French lentils, dried

2 cloves garlic, crushed

1 yellow onion, chopped

400g tomato sauce (organic)

2 tbsp. extra virgin olive oil

1 tsp dried (basil, thyme and oregano)

2 cups of water

Kosher salt and freshly ground black pepper to taste

Directions:

Combine the lentils and water in a pot and bring to a boil over medium-high heat. Once the water starts boiling, lower the heat and simmer for about 30 minutes until the lentils are tender.

While the lentils are cooking, place a medium skillet over medium heat and pour in 1 tablespoon of oil and cook the onions for 5 minutes till they become soft, then add the garlic and sauté for 1-2 minutes.

Stir in the dried herbs, tomato sauce, salt and pepper and simmer for about 20 minutes until the sauce is thick.

Now add cooked lentils to the sauce and simmer for 10 more minutes

Meanwhile, pour the remaining olive oil in a medium pan and sauté the zoodles for about 8 minutes or until they become tender.

Serve the noodles on four plates and top with marinara. Enjoy!

Squash Spaghetti with Grilled Chicken and Avocado Sauce

Ingredients:

2-3 cups spiralized squash

1 cup grilled chicken, chopped or shredded

1 avocado, pitted

2 cloves garlic, crushed

2 tbsp. coconut milk

2 tbsp. olive oil

2 tbsp. lemon juice

¼ cup sun-dried tomatoes packed in oil

Handful of fresh basil

Kosher salt and freshly ground pepper to taste

Directions:

Combine avocado, garlic, coconut milk, lemon juice, basil, salt and pepper in a food processor and pulse until they become smooth.

Pour a bit of olive oil in a medium skillet over medium heat and sauté the squash spaghetti until desired tenderness is achieved for about 8 minutes. Stir in the avocado sauce, tomatoes and chicken until they are well combined. Cook until heated through. Add some water if the sauce is too thick. Turn off the heat and garnish with chopped basil.

Serve immediately and enjoy!

Yummy Chicken Tetrazzini

Ingredients:

800g chicken strips

2 cups shiitake mushrooms, sliced

7 zucchini, peeled and spiralized

1 ½ cups frozen peas

4 cloves garlic, finely chopped

½ cup red onion, finely chopped

1 cup almond flour

100ml coconut milk

4 tbsp. organic butter

½ cup red wine

1 tbsp. arrowroot powder

1 tbsp. fresh thyme, finely chopped

Kosher salt +freshly ground black pepper to taste

Chopped fresh parsley, for topping

Directions:

Liberally season the chicken strips with salt and pepper. Place a large sauté pan over high heat and melt half the butter. Brown the seasoned chicken strips and transfer to a large platter.

Add the remaining butter to the same pan and sauté the onions, garlic and mushroom all together until tender and lightly browned. Stir in the coconut milk, thyme and wine and allow simmering for 5-10 minutes until thick. If the sauce takes long to thicken, combine the arrowroot powder with a little water and add to the pan.

Now stir in the peas and turn off the heat. Combine the chicken strips, zoodles and the vegetable mixture and toss well to combine. Scoop this into a casserole dish and set aside.

Now mix the almond flour with 2 tablespoons of butter and a good pinch of kosher salt in a food processor. Pulse until crumbly. Spread this crumble over the casserole dish.

Turn you oven on to 356 F and bake for 30 minutes.

Remove the casserole from the oven and let stand for 10 minutes, then garnish with fresh parsley. Serve immediately.

Zucchini Tuna Casserole

Ingredients:

3 small zucchini, spiralized

1 celery stalk, chopped

2 cans tuna

3 cloves garlic, minced

1 onion, chopped

1 tbsp. arrowroot powder

3 tbsp. organic ghee

1 can coconut milk

Pink sea salt and freshly cracked black pepper to taste

Directions:

Start by pre-heating your oven to 347 F.

Pour 1 tablespoon of ghee in a medium skillet over medium heat. Sauté the celery, onion and garlic. Stir in the salt and pepper and cook until the veggies become golden for about 7 minutes.

Mix the remaining ghee with the arrowroot powder over low heat until bubbly, then season with salt and pepper. Stir in the coconut milk and simmer until it becomes thick for about 8 minutes.

Pour the tuna into a bowl and mash it up using a fork and combine it with the celery mixture and the zoodles. Transfer this to a casserole dish and pour the coconut mixture over the casserole. Bake for 1 hour and remove from oven. Let it stand for 10 minutes and serve immediately.

Desserts

Savory Desserts

Baked Beet Chips with Tzatziki

Ingredients

5 beets, peeled and very thinly sliced

3 tbsp. palm oil

Coarse sea salt

Tzatziki:

1 ¼ cups coconut yogurt

¾ cup cucumber, peeled and minced finely

1 clove garlic, minced

½ tbsp. fresh parsley, minced

½ tbsp. dill

½ tbsp. chives, minced

½ tbsp. fresh mint leaves, minced

1 tsp freshly squeezed lemon juice

½ tsp coarse sea salt

Freshly ground pepper

Directions

Start by preheating your oven to 325 F and line a rimmed baking sheet with parchment paper

Lay out the sliced beets on a paper towel, to absorb most of the moisture so they can cook faster.

Transfer the sliced beets on the baking sheet and liberally coat with palm oil or your favorite oil. Use your hands to ensure all the slices are well coated.

Lightly grease another baking sheet and place it over the beets, this will help them cook flat and evenly.

Bake the sliced beets for about 20 minutes at center rack, rotating halfway through. Remove the top baking sheet and bake uncovered for another 10 minutes until slightly browned.

Remove from oven and let cool and become crisp.

Tzatziki:

Combine all the ingredients until you get an even consistency. If it's too thick, add a little water to thin. Serve as a dip for the beet chips. Enjoy!

Mango Spiced Chicken Wings

Ingredients

24 pieces chicken wings

1 onion, chopped

2 mangoes, peeled and chopped

3 tbsp. red palm oil

1 red bell pepper, chopped

½ cup apple cider vinegar

2 cloves garlic

1 tsp chipotle powder

½ cup water

Freshly ground pepper

Directions

Preheat your oven to 425 F.

Rub the wings with pepper and salt and lay them on a baking sheet. Bake for about 40 minutes until the skin start getting crisp.

Meanwhile, melt the oil in a skillet and sauté the onions, pepper and garlic for 8 minutes until soft.

Stir in the mangoes, water and vinegar and bring to a boil. Now lower heat and let simmer for 15minutes until mangoes are really soft.

Puree the sauce in your blender and return to the pan. Season with the chipotle powder, pepper and a bit of salt.

Remove the baking sheet from oven and pour about ¾ of the sauce over the wings and toss well to coat. Return the wings in the oven under broil mode and broil until they start browning.

Remove from oven and serve hot. Drizzle with the remaining mango sauce. Enjoy!

Seitan Bacon-Avocado stuffed Peppers

Ingredients

450g sweet baby peppers

150g Seitan bacon, chopped

2 ripe avocados

1 tbsp. hot sauce

2 tbsp. freshly squeezed lime juice

½ bunch cilantro, chopped

Coarse sea salt

Directions

Preheat your oven to 350 F.

Cut the peppers in half, lengthwise, removing the seeds and membrane. Arrange them in a baking sheet and lightly spray with cooking spray and bake for 10 minutes.

As the peppers are baking, mash up the avocado in a bowl and combine with the hot sauce, lime juice, salt and the cilantro and sauté the Seitan bacon in a skillet until they become crisp and browned.

Use a spoon to scoop the avocado mash into the peppers and top with Seitan bacon bits. Enjoy!

Roasted pumpkin seeds

Ingredients

Scrape out the seed and pulp from 1 or 2 pumpkins

Garlic salt

¼ cup salt

2-3 tbsp. olive oil

Directions

Soak the pulp and seeds in a bowl of water with the ¼ cup salt. Let stand for 2 days.

After the 2 days, separate the seeds from the pulp and set your oven to 325 F.

Rinse the seeds and pat dry with paper towels then sprinkle with garlic salt and coat with the olive oil. Line a baking sheet with parchment paper and spread out the seeds. Roast for 20 minutes until they start browning. Remove from oven and let cool slightly. Enjoy!

Yummy Broiled Tomato

Ingredients

5 Roma tomatoes, sliced

Freshly ground pepper

Olive oil

Coarse sea salt

Directions

Preheat your broiler and prepare your baking sheet by lining it with parchment paper.

Toss the tomato slices with salt, pepper and olive oil. Arrange them in a single layer and broil for 7 minutes until they start getting crisp. Remove from broiler and let cool a bit. Enjoy!

Sweet Desserts

Barbequed Peaches & Plum with Cream Cheese

Ingredients:

10 ripe peaches, cut in halves and pitted

24 purple/ red plums cut in halves and pitted, with 4 sliced thinly

2 tbsp. freshly squeezed lemon juice

1 cup water

½ cup raw honey

6 tbsp. organic butter, melted

Cream cheese for serving

Directions:

Prepare your grill and set to medium heat.

Meanwhile, place a medium saucepan over medium to high heat and add the water, sliced plums and ¾ cup of honey. Once it starts boiling, cover and bring to a gentle simmer for 10 minutes. The plums should be super soft. Place the cooked plums in your food processor and pulse until it forms a smooth puree. Scoop the puree into a small bowl and combine with lemon juice.

Now, whisk the melted butter with the remaining honey and set aside. Grill the peaches and plums over medium heat until desired tenderness is achieved, that's about 6 minutes. Baste the fruits with the butter-honey paste and turn them once on the grill. Keep grilling until they caramelize and char slightly say about 2 more minutes.

Serve the grilled fruits on fruit bowls and drizzle with the plum puree. Top with a generous dollop of cream cheese and enjoy!

Grilled Pineapple Sundaes with Shredded Coconut

Ingredients:

1 whole ripe pineapple. Peeled, cored and cut in rings

½ cup shredded coconut, sweetened

2 tsp vegetable oil

Frozen vanilla yogurt, fat free

Mint sprigs

Directions:

Prepare a grill and set to medium. Lightly brush the pineapple rings with vegetable oil and place on the grill. Turn the pineapples once or twice and grill until they are soft and a bit charred, for about 8 minutes. Transfer the pineapples to a cutting board and chop them up.

Now toast the shredded coconut in a small pan over low heat and serve on a plate.

Serve the fro-yo (frozen yogurt) into sundae glasses or ice cream bowl and place the grilled pineapple on top, sprinkle with toasted coconut and garnish with mint sprigs. Serve immediately.

BBQ Berry Crostini with Crème Fraiche

Ingredients:

4 cups fresh mixed berries

3-4 slices original country bread, cut in half cross-wise

1/8 cup pure maple syrup

1 tbsp. natural honey

Organic unsalted butter, softened for brushing

½ cup paleo crème fraiche

A good pinch kosher salt

Directions:

Start by lighting an outdoor charcoal fire grill.

Combine honey with crème fraiche in a small bowl and whisk thoroughly until they are well blended.

Butter both sides of the bread slices and spread with a bit of maple syrup. Grill the bread over medium heat until it is caramelized and crisp for about 3 minutes. Remove from grill and place on a plate to cool off.

Place the berries in a mixing bowl and toss with kosher salt and maple syrup. Line the berries on a grill basket or if you don't have one, on a perforated grill pan/ sheet and then grill over medium heat, tossing frequently until they start bursting, that should be about 4-5 minutes. Remove from grill and transfer to a bowl.

Top the crostini with warm berries and with generous dollops of honeyed crème fraiche. Enjoy!

Spiralized Pear, Figs and Honeyed Walnuts

Ingredients:

2 pears, spiralized into pretty ribbons

½ cup walnuts

6-8 black mission figs, cut in halves

1/3 tsp vanilla extract

1 tbsp. raw honey and more for drizzling

½ cup ricotta cheese

Directions

Pre-heat your oven to 365 F and line 2 baking dishes with parchment paper. Place the figs on one dish and use your index finger the sliced sides with honey and bake for 10 minutes. On the second dish, place the walnuts and toss with honey using your hands. Bake the walnuts for 3 minutes and remove them from the oven. Transfer the figs and walnuts to a medium bowl.

Whip up the cheese using your food processor and transfer to a small bowl. Combine with vanilla extract and honey until they are well blended.

Arrange the pear ribbons on a plate as the base for your desert and top with the nuts and the figs, creating a circle then sprinkle the sweetened ricotta and a few of the nuts and figs.

Minty Cucumber Popsicles

Ingredients:

1 cucumber, spirallized

¾ cup lime juice, freshly squeezed

4 tbsp. fresh mint, chopped

Water

Directions:

Prepare 6 Popsicle molds and in each, place 2 teaspoons of the chopped mint followed by 2 tablespoons of lime juice. Add 2-3 tablespoons of the noodles and top with a bit of water and secure the mold.

Freeze the popsicles for a minimum of 4 hours but preferably overnight.

Before indulging in your Popsicle, run the mold under some warm water first.

Enjoy!

Apple Cider Cocktail

Ingredients:

1 apple, peeled and spiralized

120ml apple cider

30ml St. Germaine

80ml red wine

3 ice cubes

Directions:

Combine all the contents apart from the apple spirals in a cocktail mixer and shake well.

Pour into a tall glass and garnish with apple spirals.

Candy bars

Ingredients

¼ cup cocoa powder

¼ cup ground almonds

¼ cup ground hazelnuts

¾ cup shredded coconut, unsweetened

3 tbsp. coconut oil

1 tbsp. raw honey

Directions

Place a medium saucepan over low-medium heat and add the honey and coconut oil. Remove from heat as soon as the two melt into each other to avoid burning.

Stir in the ground nuts, cocoa powder and shredded coconut to the honey mixture and combine well.

Transfer this mixture into a baking sheet that is lined with parchment paper and allow to cool. Once cooled, form desired shapes then chill in the fridge for 4 hours or more.

Enjoy!

Healthy Berry Ice Cream

Ingredients

500g frozen strawberries, unsweetened

420 ml coconut milk

½ tbsp. freshly squeezed lemon juice

1/tsp stevia extract

Directions

Combine all the ingredients in your food processor and pulse until the strawberries are smooth. You can eat it instantly otherwise if you want to eat it later, freeze but take it out 30 minutes before eating because it will be frozen rock-hard due to the lack of sugar.

Enjoy!

CONCLUSION

Thank you again for downloading this book!

I hope this book was able to help you understand what ketogenic diet is and how to jumpstart a healthier lifestyle.

If you haven't started yet, make that decision today. Remember, being healthy is a decision. The ketogenic diet might be very different from what you are used to, and you may have to say goodbye to your favorite comfort food, but give it a chance, see what it can do to your overall health, weight loss process and even disposition, and you will be amazed on how effective it is in achieving your goals.

In addition, the next time that you hear diet, do not automatically feel restricted, but instead view it as choosing the right and healthy food for you. It does not also mean that you will be saying goodbye to mouth-watering dishes, but with the keto diet, there are actually hundreds of dishes and alternatives to choose from. This is why planning your meals and researching will do wonders to make your diet journey a less bumpy ones.

There are chances that you will feel that you have failed or gave in to the temptation of consuming non-keto food, but then again, life is also about chances. Learn from that mistake, and start all over again.

I challenge you to first try this diet for 21 days, as your new healthy habit is in place, it will actually become more and more easy for you to make ketogenic diet not as a weight loss tool but as an entirely lifestyle change. Make that decision now! A happier and healthier you is just around the corner with ketodiet.

Finally, if you enjoyed this book, then I'd like to ask you for a favor, would you be kind enough to leave a review for this book on Amazon? It'd be greatly appreciated!

Click here to leave a review for this book on Amazon!

Thank you and good luck!

CHECK OUT MY OTHER BOOKS

Below you'll find some of my other popular books that are popular on Amazon and Kindle as well. Simply click on the links below to check them out. Alternatively, you can visit my author page on Amazon to see other work done by me.

If the links do not work, for whatever reason, you can simply search for these titles on the Amazon website to find them.

BOOKS BY LR SMITH:

Low Carb High Fat - Click here

Anti-Inflammatory Diet - Click here

Mediterranean Diet - Click here

Whole Food - Click here

Dash Diet - Click here

Bone Broth - Click here

www.ingramcontent.com/pod-product-compliance
Lightning Source LLC
Chambersburg PA
CBHW062158280526
45788CB00001B/350